Curing
Fibromyalgia
Naturally

with
Chinese
Medicine

Bob Flaws

BLUE POPPY PRESS

Published by:
BLUE POPPY PRESS
A Division of Blue Poppy Enterprises, Inc.
3450 Penrose Place, Suite 110
BOULDER, CO 80301

First Edition, February 2000

ISBN 1-891845-09-8   LC# 99 75599
COPYRIGHT 2000 © BLUE POPPY PRESS

All rights reserved. No part of this book may be reproduced, stored in a retrieval system, transcribed in any form or by any means, electronic, mechanical, photocopy, recording, or any other means, or translated into any language without the prior written permission of the publisher.

WARNING: When following some of the self-care techniques given in this book, failure to follow the author's instruction may result in side effects or negative reactions. Therefore, please be sure to follow the author's instructions carefully for all self-care techniques and modalities. For instance, wrong or excessive application of moxibustion may cause local burns with redness, inflammation, blistering, or even possible scarring. If you have any questions about doing these techniques safely and without unwanted side effects, please see a local professional practitioner for instruction.

DISCLAIMER: The information in this book is given in good faith. However, the author and the publishers cannot be held responsible for any error or omission. The publishers will not accept liabilities for any injuries or damages caused to the reader that may result from the reader's acting upon or using the content contained in this book.

COMP Designation: Original work using a standard translational terminology

Printed at Johnson Printing in Boulder, CO
on essentially chlorine-free paper
Cover design by Jeff Fuller, Crescent Moon

10 9 8 7 6 5 4 3 2 1

Preface

Fibromyalgia is a mysteriously debilitating syndrome. Although it does not involve any physical damage to the body, it is characterized by such severe, widespread pain that it is often incapacitating. As if that were not enough, the symptoms of fibromyalgia also include chronic muscle stiffness, insomnia, depression, and fatigue. This condition is often mistaken for chronic fatigue syndrome (CFS), and there is no single laboratory test to determine its presence. Therefore, many sufferers of fibromyalgia bounce from doctor to doctor seeking diagnosis and relief which, all too often, elude them.

Happily, traditional Chinese medicine has been treating muscle pain and stiffness, insomnia, depression, and fatigue for not less than a historically verified and recorded 2,000 years. Although the diagnostic label of fibromyalgia maybe relatively new, there is nothing new or unusual about this disease for Chinese doctors. Using a combination of no or low cost home remedies as well as the safe and effective professional treatments of Chinese medicine, it is my experience that the overwhelming majority of fibromyalgia sufferers can find substantial relief from all these ills by using the age-old wisdom of Chinese medicine. The good news is, not only is Chinese medicine able to treat this condition, when it does, it does so without *any* side effects. In addition, Chinese medicine teaches a person how to take back control over their own health, restoring the power to be well to each individual.

If you or someone you know suffers from fibromyalgia, then this book is for you. Although I am a Chinese medical gynecologist, three times or more women suffer from fibromyalgia than men. Therefore, I have seen a lot of fibromyalgia over the years. In fact, I have practiced Chinese medicine for over 20 years in Asia,

Europe, and America and I know Chinese medicine can help you.

Bob Flaws
Boulder, CO
August 1999

Table of Contents

1
Introduction

Hannah is beside herself and doesn't know what to do. Her body has been aching all over for several months. In addition, she has been extremely fatigued and depressed. If she could only get a good night's sleep, she thinks she might feel better. However, she can only sleep till four o'clock each night. Then she lies awake in her bed, tossing and turning, unable to go back to sleep. Her PMS has gotten so bad lately that she's afraid her husband is going to leave her, and if she misses any more work, her boss is certainly going to fire her. To top it off, every time she eats, her abdomen becomes bloated and crampy and she has urgent diarrhea several times per day. She's been to several different doctors and all have told her she has something else. One tested her for rheumatoid arthritis and lupus erythamotosus which, thankfully, turned out to be negative. Another told her she was depressed. A third said she had something called chronic fatigue syndrome and that she may be sick for months and even years. She's been taking Ibuprofen as if it were M & M's™. One of the doctors prescribed Prozac, but she didn't want to take it. Another prescribed Flexeril, but she finds it makes her so drowsy, she can't concentrate or think. If she doesn't find a solution to all this soon, Hannah thinks she really will go crazy.

If this sounds like you or anyone you know, read on. What Hannah really has is fibromyalgia, along with 3-6 million other Americans,[1] and it is the causes and cure of fibromyalgia that are the subjects of this book.

---

[1] "What is Fibromyalgia," www.futureone.com/~hunter/what.htm, p. 1

What is fibromyalgia?

Fibromyalgia, also called fibromyalgia syndrome or FMS, is a condition mostly affecting women between 20-50 years of age. It is characterized by chronic, widespread, severe muscular aching, pain, and stiffness accompanied by insomnia, fatigue, and depression. Unlike osteoarthritis, rheumatoid arthritis, and lupus erythamotosus, it is neither a rheumatic, inflammatory, progressive, or degenerative disorder. However, it is also not solely a psychosomatic or psychiatric disorder. In other words, it is not all in the patient's head. What it is is a chronic, debilitating condition of unknown etiology or cause, but which is probably caused by a number of different factors involving a complex relationship between the psyche (the mind) and the soma (the body). In 1987, the American Medical Association (AMA) recognized FMS as a true illness and major cause of disability.[2]

Because this condition does not result in any physical damage to the body or its tissues, there is no one laboratory test or x-ray which can confirm this diagnosis. Because this condition is so commonly associated with chronic, enduring fatigue, it is often confused with chronic fatigue syndrome (CFS) or what is also known as chronic fatigue immune deficiency syndrome (CFIDS) in the U.S. However, unlike CFS, fibromyalgia sufferers usually experience much more significant muscle-joint aching and pain. It is estimated that as much as 75% of CFS-diagnosed patients actually fit the criteria for FMS.[3] Fibromyalgia can also be differentiated from other chronic muscle-joint pain by the presence of pain or tenderness upon pressure in at least 11 out of

---

[2] Starlanyl, Devin J., "FMS: Fibromyalgia Syndrome," www.sover.net/~devstar/fmsdef.htm, p. 1

[3] "What is Fibromyalgia?," *op. cit.*, p. 1

18 specific points on the body.[4] In addition to the above characteristics, FMS sufferers are also typically hypersensitive to odors, bright lights, and loud noises. Headaches and jaw pain, also known as temporomandibular joint (TMJ) pain, are common.

The clinical features of FMS

The word syndrome in fibromyalgia syndrome means that this condition presents with a varying range of accompanying signs and symptoms besides just muscle and joint aching and pain. Although Western medicine cannot explain why these symptoms occur together as they do, Western doctors do recognize this constellation of symptoms as a clinical entity or disease. In Western medicine, groups of commonly occurring symptoms of unknown causes are called syndromes. Therefore, because FMS is a syndrome, it means that patients with this condition display a number of different signs and symptoms. Some of these are listed below along with the rates of their occurrence.

90-100% of FMS sufferers have:

Generalized body pain effecting all four quadrants of the body
Fatigue
Muscular stiffness

These three symptoms are all typically worse in the morning. FMS patients often say their arms and legs feel "like tied to concrete blocks." The muscular pain associated with FMS is described as deep, burning, throbbing, shooting, and/or stabbing. And the fatigue may range from simple, random exhaustion to being unable to get out of bed.

---

[4] It was the Copenhagen Declaration published in 1990 that established the diagnostic criteria of pressure pain at a minimum of 11 of 18 specific points on the body.

70-90% of FMS sufferers will also have one or more of the following:

Post-exertional malaise
Sleep disturbances
Headaches, either migraine or tension
Tenderness to pressure at certain, specific spots on the body
Swollen feet
Numbness and/or tingling
Difficulty thinking and concentrating, a.k.a. "brain fog"
Dizziness
Sensitivity to light, noise, and/or smells
Hypersensitivity to stress
Dysmenorrhea or painful menstruation
Dry mouth

In terms of sleep disturbances, FMS sufferers are usually able to fall asleep but then are not able to sleep soundly or wake up too early in the morning. In terms of the swollen feet, the feet may actually be swollen or they may only feel swollen to the patient. The dizziness of FMS is often orthostatic hypotension, meaning dizziness when standing up. Dysmenorrhea may also be diagnosed as endometriosis.

50-70% of FMS sufferers will also have one or more of the following:

Irritable bowel syndrome (IBS)
Blurred vision
Mood swings
Heart palpitations
Cold extremities
Feverish feelings
Allergies

Irritable bowel syndrome refers to a constellation of symptoms including lower abdominal bloating, cramping, and pain, typically after eating, diarrhea and/or constipation, and mucus in the stools. It is sometimes also referred to as mucus colitis or allergic colitis. Based on my own clinical experience, I would add the words "night blindness" after blurred vision. Many women with this condition have decreased visual acuity at night which makes them reluctant or uncomfortable to drive at night even if, strictly speaking, they do not have the Western medical disease of nyctalopia or night blindness.

15-50% of FMS sufferers will also have one or more of the following:

Restless leg syndrome
Muscle twitches
Itchy skin
Hearing disturbances
Night sweats
Breathing problems
Proneness to infections
Skin rashes
Interstitial cystitis
TMJ
Multiple chemical sensitivities

Restless leg syndrome refers to a vague, hard to describe feeling of discomfort experienced in the legs, usually at night, characterized by the need to constantly move the legs in order to try and relieve this discomfort. Breathing problems include allergic rhinitis and allergic asthma. Interstitial cystitis is characterized by decreased urinary capacity and, therefore, frequent, painful urination and hematuria. Typically, this condition effects middle-aged women and may be either an allergic or autoimmune disease. Multiple chemical sensitivities are also referred to as environmental illness.

Less than 15% of FMS sufferers also display major depression. However, most FMS sufferers are mildly depressed. Other symptoms or conditions also reported in the FMS literature and which I have seen in a number of patients in my own practice are new or worsening PMS, fibrocystic breast disease (FBD), and mouth sores.

In order to qualify for a diagnosis of fibromyalgia, the above generalized muscle pain, stiffness, and fatigue have to have lasted for not less than three months. In addition, as stated above, at least 11 out of 18 specific tender points on the body should be painful to palpation.

How Western medicine treats fibromyalgia

Because fibromyalgia involves a number of different symptoms, Western physicians try to treat this disorder by prescribing various medications and treatments for each of these different symptoms. In other words, because it has not yet identified the underlying cause of FMS, Western medicine has no single treatment for FMS *per se.* This means that antidepressants, such as Prozac, Elavil, Paxil, and Xanax, are commonly prescribed to treat the sleep and mood, while non-steroidal anti-inflammatories (NSAIDS), such as Ibuprofen, are prescribed for the pain. In addition, trigger points, *i.e.,* points that are hypersensitive to pressure, may be injected with lidocaine, a local anesthetic. Many FMS patients benefit from regular weekly massages, but few insurance companies will pay for this even when prescribed by an MD.

Unfortunately, not all patients tolerate antidepressants such as Prozac, Elavil, and Paxil without side effects. For instance, the side effects of Prozac include skin rashes, hives, and itching, headache, nervousness, insomnia, drowsiness and fatigue, tremors, dizziness, and impaired concentration.[5] In addition, many other patients simply do not want to take such Western

---

[5] Long, James W., *The Essential Guide to Prescription Drugs*, Harper & Row, NY, 1990, p. 483

psychotropic pharmaceuticals. NSAIDS can be very effective for acute pain relief, but they also have their own potential side effects, such as skin rashes, hives, and itching, headache, dizziness, blurred vision, ringing in the ears, depression, mouth sores, and gastrointestinal upset.[6] Ironically, some of these side effects include many of the symptoms of FMS. There are also some concerns about NSAIDS' effect on the kidneys when taken over a prolonged period of time.[7] Unfortunately, when used in the treatment of fibromyalgia, NSAIDS usually do have to be taken for such a prolonged time.

The good news

The good news is that traditional Chinese medicine treats all the above signs and symptoms associated with fibromyalgia syndrome very effectively and *without side effects.* In addition, Chinese medicine can explain the disease causes and disease mechanisms at work in each fibromyalgia sufferer's own personal case. Further, Chinese medicine treats the underlying root causes of fibromyalgia. It does not just palliate its symptoms.

East is East and West is West

In order for the reader to understand and make sense of the rest of this book on Chinese medicine and fibromyalgia, one must understand that Chinese medicine is a distinct and separate system of medical thought and practice from modern Western medicine. This means that one must shift models of reality when it comes to thinking about Chinese medicine. It has taken the Chinese more than 2,000 years to develop this medical system. In fact, Chinese medicine is the oldest continually practiced, literate, professional medicine in the world. As such one cannot

---

[6] *Ibid.*, p. 538

[7] Ronco, P. & Flahault, A., "Drug-induced End Stage Renal Disease," *New England Journal of Medicine*, Vol. 331, #25, 1994, p. 1711-1712

understand Chinese medicine by trying to explain it in Western scientific or medical terms.

Most people reading this book have probably taken high school biology back when they were sophomores. Whether we recognize it or not, most of us Westerners think of what we learned about the human body in high school as "the really real" description of reality, not one possible description. However, if Chinese medicine is to make any sense to Westerners at all, one must be able to entertain the notion that there are potentially other valid descriptions of the human body, its functions, health, and disease. In grappling with this fundamentally important issue, it is useful to think about the concepts of a map and the terrain it describes.

If we take the United States of America as an example, we can have numerous different maps of this country's land mass. One map might show population. Another might show per capita incomes. Another might show religious or ethnic distributions. Yet another might be a road map. And still another might be a map showing political, *i.e.*, state boundaries. In fact, there could be an infinite number of potentially different maps of the United States depending on what one was trying to show and do. As long as the map is based on accurate information and has been created with self-consistent logic, then one map is not necessarily more correct than another. The issue is to use the right map for what you are trying to do. If one wants to drive from Chicago to Washington DC, then a road map is probably the right one *for that job* but is not necessarily a truer or "more real" description of the United States than a map showing annual rainfall.

What I am getting at here is that *the map is not the terrain*. The Western biological map of the human body is only one potentially useful medical map. It is no more true than the traditional Chinese medical map, and the "facts" of one map cannot be reduced to the criteria or standards of another *unless they share the same logic right from the beginning*. As long as the Western medical map is capable of solving a person's disease in a cost-effective, time-efficient manner without side effects or iatrogenesis (meaning doctor-caused disease), then it is a useful map. Chinese medicine needs to be judged in the same way. The Chinese medical map of health and disease is just as "real" as the Western biological map as long as, using it, professional practitioners are able to solve their patients' health problems in a safe and effective way.

Therefore, the following chapter is an introduction to the basics of Chinese medicine. Unless one understands some of the fundamental theories and "facts" of Chinese medicine, one will not be able to understand or accept the reasons for some of the Chinese medical treatments of fibromyalgia. As the reader will quickly see from this brief overview of Chinese medicine, "This doesn't look like Kansas, Toto!"

2

An Introduction to the Basic Concepts of Chinese Medicine

As we have seen in the preceding chapter, fibromyalgia is actually a syndrome made up of several different major symptoms. The four most important of these in my experience are generalized body pain, insomnia, fatigue, and mild depression. Each of these four is a traditional Chinese disease category in its own right. Therefore, if you were to ask what is the traditional Chinese disease categories covering the modern Western disease of fibromyalgia, the answer would be *bi zheng* or impediment condition, *bu mian* or insomnia, *xu lao* or vacuity taxation (*i.e.*, chronic, severe fatigue), and *yu zheng*, depression. By combining the Chinese understandings and diagnosis of these four key traditional Chinese diseases, we can easily understand the modern disease of fibromylagia syndrome.

Of these four, bodily pain is the single most important, defining characteristic of fibromylagia as opposed to chronic fatigue syndrome. The Chinese medical term for all diseases whose main symptom is muscle-joint pain is *bi zheng*. This translates as "impediment condition." In Chinese medicine, *bi* or impediment means a blockage or obstruction that results in pain. A number of questions come to mind from this statement. What is being blocked or obstructed? How does this blockage or obstruction come about? And, probably the most important question, especially for people suffering with fibromyalgia, what can be done to reduce or eliminate this pain? Other important questions are what is the relationship between this body pain and insomnia, fatigue, and depression and why do these three conditions occur together with this bodily pain? And further, why is fibromyalgia so commonly seen in women and not so commonly in men? The remainder of this book will help you see how Chinese medicine answers these questions.

To understand how traditional Chinese medicine answers the above questions and treats the constellation of conditions we now refer to as FMS, we first need to discuss, describe, and explain the fundamental concepts of this oldest professionally practiced, literate, holistic medical system. As a system, Chinese medicine is logical. Based on its theories, a practitioner can perform treatments that achieve the desired effect. Therefore, it is also pragmatic and scientific in its own way. However, Chinese medicine is a separate system from modern Western medicine, and, as such, cannot be explained by Western medical words or logic. In other words, to truly understand the how and why of Chinese medicine, we need to approach it on its own terms.

When first hearing the theories and concepts of Chinese medicine, the reader may find them odd and mystifying. This is only natural when we begin to look at something that not only *appears different* but *is completely different than what we have been raised to believe as true and real.* As I tell my patients, if reality is what the vast majority of people agree to be true, then the Chinese medical view of the body and what causes disease must be "true and real." Over one billion people in Asia view the body and disease according to the ideas of Chinese medicine. However, more importantly, the fact that Chinese medicine has been effectively treating all four of the major conditions defining FMS for over 2,000 years is what gives these ideas truth and reality.

Yin & yang

Yin and yang are the cornerstones for understanding, diagnosing, and treating the body and mind in Chinese medicine. In a sense, all the other theories and concepts of Chinese medicine are nothing other than an elaboration of yin and yang. Most people have probably already heard of yin and yang but may have only a fuzzy idea of what these terms mean.

The concepts of yin and yang can be used to describe everything that exists in the universe, including all the parts and functions of the body. Originally, yin referred to the shady side of a hill and yang to the sunny side of the hill. Since sunshine and shade are two interdependent sides of a single reality, these two aspects of the hill are seen as part of a single whole. Other examples of yin and yang are that night exists only in relation to day and cold exists only in relation to heat. According to Chinese thought, every single thing that exists in the universe has these two aspects, a yin and a yang. Thus everything has a front and a back, a top and a bottom, a left and a right, and a beginning and an end. However, a thing is yin or yang *only in relation to its paired complement.* Nothing is in itself yin or yang.

It is the concepts of yin and yang which make Chinese medicine a holistic medicine. This is because, based on this unitary and

YIN	YANG
form	function
organs	bowels
blood	qi
inside	outside
front of body	back of body
right side	left side
lower body	upper body
cool, cold	warm, hot
stillness	activity, movement

complementary vision of reality, no body part or body function is viewed as separate or isolated from the whole person. The table above shows a partial list of yin and yang pairs as they apply to the body. However, it is important to remember that each item listed is either yin or yang only in relation to its complementary partner. Nothing is absolutely and all by itself either yin or yang. As we can see from the above list, it is possible to describe every aspect of the body in terms of yin and yang.

Qi

Qi (pronounced chee) and blood are the two most important complementary pairs of yin and yang within the human body. It is said that, in the world, yin and yang are water and fire, but, in the human body, yin and yang are blood and qi. Qi is yang in relation to blood which is yin. Qi is often translated as energy and definitely energy is a manifestation of qi. Chinese language scholars would say, however, that qi is larger than any single type of energy described by modern Western science. Paul Unschuld, perhaps the greatest living sinologist, translates the word qi as influences. This conveys the sense that qi is what is responsible for change and movement. Thus, within Chinese medicine, qi is that which motivates all movement and transformation or change.

In Chinese medicine, qi is defined as having five specific functions:

1. Defense

It is qi which is responsible for protecting the exterior of the body from invasion by external pathogens. This qi, called defensive qi, flows through the exterior portion of the body. The defensive qi plays an extremely important role in the development and the prevention of impediment conditions. As we shall see, when this qi is weak, external pathogens can enter and lodge in the body, especially in the joints, creating the blockage and obstruction that then develop into impediment conditions. In addition, people who are prone to infections or who have allergies typically have weak defensive qi.

2. Transformation

Qi transforms substances so that they can be utilized by the body. An example of this function is the transformation of the food we eat into nutrients to nourish the body, thus producing more qi and blood.

3. Warmth

Qi, being relatively yang, is inherently warm. One of the main functions of the qi is to warm the entire body, both inside and out. If this warming function of the qi is weak, cold may cause the flow of qi and blood to slow and congeal similar to the way cold effects water to produce ice.

4. Restraint

It is qi which holds all the organs and substances in their proper place. Thus all the organs, blood, and fluids need qi to keep them from falling or leaking out of their specific pathways. If this function of qi is weak, then problems like uterine prolapse, easy bruising, or urinary incontinence may occur.

5. Transportation

Qi provides the motivating force for all transportation in the body. Every aspect of the body that moves is moved by the qi. Hence the qi moves the blood and body fluids throughout the body. It is also qi which moves food through the stomach and the blood through its vessels.

Blood

In Chinese medicine, blood refers to the red fluid that flows through our vessels as recognized in modern Western medicine, but it also has meanings and implications which are different from those of modern Western medicine. Most basically, blood is that substance which nourishes and moistens all the body tissues. Without blood, no body tissue can function properly. In addition, when blood is insufficient or scanty, tissue becomes dry and withers.

Qi and blood are closely interrelated. It is said that, "Qi is the commander of the blood, and blood is the mother of qi." This means that it is qi which moves the blood but that it is the blood which provides the nourishment and physical foundation for the creation and existence of the qi.

In Chinese medicine, blood provides the following functions for the body:

1. Nourishment

Blood nourishes the body. Along with qi, the blood goes to every part of the body. When the blood is insufficient, function decreases and tissue atrophies or shrinks.

2. Moistening

Blood moistens the body tissues. This includes the skin, eyes, and ligaments and tendons of the body. Thus blood insufficiency can cause drying out and consequent stiffening of various tissues throughout the body.

3. Blood provides the material foundation for the spirit or mind.

In Chinese medicine, the mind and body are not two separate things. The spirit is nothing other than a great accumulation of qi. The blood (yin) supplies the material support and nourishment for the spirit (yang) so that it accumulates, becomes bright, and stays rooted in the body. If the blood becomes insufficient, the mind can "float," causing problems like insomnia, agitation, and unrest.

16

Essence

Along with qi and blood, essence is one of the three most important constituents of the body. Essence is the most fundamental material the body utilizes for its growth, maturation, and reproduction. There are two forms of this essence. We inherit essence from our parents and also produce our own essence from the food we eat, the liquids we drink, and the air we breathe.

The essence which comes from our parents is what determines our basic constitution, strength, and vitality. We each have a finite, limited amount of this inherited essence. It is important to protect and conserve this essence because all bodily functions depend upon it, and, when it is gone, we die. Thus, the depletion of essence has serious implications for our overall health and well-being. Fortunately, the essence derived from food and drink helps to bolster and support this inherited essence. This is possible if we eat healthy and do not utilize more of our qi and blood than we create each day. Then, when we sleep at night, the surplus qi and especially the blood are transformed into essence.

The viscera & bowels

In Chinese medicine, the internal organs have a wider area of function and influence than in Western medicine. Each organ has distinct responsibilities for maintaining the physical health and psychological well-being of the individual. When thinking about the internal organs according to Chinese medicine it is more accurate to view an organ as a network that spreads throughout the body, rather than as a distinct and separate physical organ as described by Western science. In Chinese medicine, the relationship between the various organs and other parts of the body is made possible by the channel and network vessel system which we will discuss below.

Because the internal organs are conceived differently and perform different functions from their same named organs in modern Western medicine, they are referred to as the viscera and bowels. This is because, in Chinese medicine, there are five main viscera which are relatively yin and six main bowels which are relatively yang. The five yin organs are the heart, lungs, liver, spleen, and kidneys. The six yang bowels are the stomach, small intestine, large intestine, gallbladder, urinary bladder, and a system that Chinese medicine refers to as the triple burner. All the functions of the entire body are subsumed or described under these eleven viscera and bowels. Thus Chinese medicine *as a system* does not "have" a pancreas, a pituitary gland, or the ovaries. Nonetheless, the functions of these Western organs are described within the Chinese medicine system of the five viscera and six bowels.

The five viscera are the most important in this system. These are the organs that Chinese medicine says are responsible for the creation and transformation of qi and blood and the storage of essence. For instance, the kidneys are responsible for the excretion of urine but are also responsible for hearing, the strength of the bones including the low back, sexual reproduction, maturation and growth. This points out that the Chinese organs may have the same name and even some overlapping functions but yet are quite different from the organs of modern Western medicine. Each of the five viscera also has a corresponding tissue, sense, spirit, and emotion related to it. These are outlined in the table below.

Organ Correspondences

Organ	Tissue	Sense	Spirit	Emotion
Kidneys	bones/ head hair	hearing	will	fear
Liver	sinews	sight	ethereal soul	anger
Spleen	flesh	taste	thought	obsession/ worry
Lungs	skin/ body hair	smell	corporeal soul	grief/ sadness
Heart	blood vessels	speech	spirit	joy/fright

In addition, each viscus or bowel possesses both a yin and a yang aspect. The yin aspect of a viscus or bowel refers to its substantial nature or tangible form. Further, an organ's yin is responsible for the nurturing, cooling, and moistening of that viscus or bowel. The yang aspect of the viscus or bowel represents its functional activities or what it does. An organ's yang aspect is also warming. These two aspects, yin and yang, form and function, cooling and heating, create good health when they are in balance. However, if either yin or yang becomes too strong or too weak, the result will be disease.

The health of all five viscera is necessary for the prevention and/or the development of rheumatic *bi* problems. However, the viscera most directly related to impediment conditions, insomnia, fatigue, and depression are the spleen, liver, heart, and kidneys. The involvement of these four viscera in fibromyalgia very dramatically illustrates the holistic nature of Chinese medicine. When these four viscera function properly and work together harmoniously, the body does not develop chronic muscle-joint pain and stiffness, we do not experience insomnia, nor are we fatigued and depressed. However, if these four viscera do not function properly, then the body is at risk to develop chronic impediment conditions, sleep disturbances, fatigue, depression, and all the other major and minor symptoms characteristic of FMS.

In the remainder of this chapter we will describe the basic functions of the spleen, liver, heart, and kidneys. In the next chapter, we will see how these four viscera specifically relate to body pain, insomnia, fatigue, and depression.

The spleen

The spleen is the single most important Chinese viscus in fibromyalgia syndrome and its dysfunction accounts for the majority of FMS symptoms. The spleen and its paired bowel, the stomach, are central in the digestive process. The spleen plays a crucial role in the body's ability to transform food and drink into qi *and* blood. In addition, the spleen, kidneys, and lungs all play

19

a part in the metabolism and movement of water throughout the body. However, the spleen plays the most crucial part when excessive body fluids gather and collect, transforming into dampness. Readers familiar with Western anatomy and physiology may be scratching their heads as they compare the Chinese medicine ideas of spleen function with what they know the spleen does from Western physiology. Again, they should be cautioned that Chinese medicine views the internal organs and their functions differently from Western medicine.

The key Chinese medical statements of fact about the spleen in terms of fibromyalgia are:

1. The spleen governs the transportation and transformation of food and water.

This means that the spleen takes the partially digested food and fluids from the stomach and begins the process of transforming it into qi, blood, and essence. Therefore, it is also said that the spleen is the source of engenderment and transformation of the qi and blood. A healthy spleen is vital for producing sufficient qi and blood. Energy and strength are both functions of the qi. Fatigue and bodily weakness are almost always symptoms of spleen vacuity weakness.

2. The spleen governs the muscles and the four limbs.

This statement is somewhat a corollary of the above statement. The muscles are dependent upon the spleen for their nourishment. If this spleen function is weak, the muscles will be weak and the legs and arms will lack power.

3. The spleen is averse to dampness.

If pathological dampness either invades the body from outside or is erroneously engendered internally, such "evil" dampness may damage and impede any or all of the spleen's functions.

4. Thought is the emotion associated with the spleen.

In the West, we do not usually think of thought as an emotion per se. Be that as it may, in Chinese medicine it is classified along with anger, joy, fear, grief, and melancholy. In particular, thinking, or perhaps I should say overthinking, causes the spleen qi to bind. This means that the spleen qi does not flow harmoniously and this typically manifests as loss of appetite, abdominal bloating after meals, and indigestion. This binding damages the spleen and eventually leads to spleen vacuity weakness. Conversely, difficulty thinking, as in "brain fog," is usually a symptom of spleen qi vacuity.

5. The spleen governs upbearing.

Upbearing is a technical term meaning the upbearing of the clear or pure part of the digestate. If this clear part is properly upborne, then the qi is engendered, the body is protected from external invasion, and especially the parts of the body located "above" the spleen, *i.e.*, the heart, lungs, and head, are all sufficiently empowered. If the spleen is too weak to upbear the clear, then the heart may become vacuous and weak, thinking may become unclear, and there may be dizziness when standing up.

The liver

The liver is the second most important viscus in Chinese medicine for understanding all the conditions associated with FMS. The basic Chinese medical statements of fact concerning the liver in terms of fibromyalgia include:

1. The liver controls coursing and discharge.

Coursing and discharge refer to the orderly spreading of qi to every part of the body. To be healthy, the qi needs to reach every part of the body. If the liver is not able to maintain the free and smooth flow of qi throughout the body, multiple physical and

21

emotional symptoms can develop. This vital function of the liver is most easily damaged by emotional causes and, in particular, by stress and frustration. When we are frustrated, our qi wants to flow but the circumstances won't allow it. In Chinese, it is said that the liver's function of coursing and discharge is damaged by unfulfilled desires, and what adult living in a civilized society can fulfill all of our desires? One of the defining characteristics of adult behavior is learning to delay the gratification of our desires. Thus, in Chinese medicine, it is said, "In adults, blame the liver." Stagnation and constraint in the flow of liver qi due to emotional frustration and stress is called liver depression qi stagnation in Chinese medicine.

Yan De-xin, a famous contemporary Chinese doctor, likes to say that, even though liver depression may not have originally caused a person's disease, if a person is chronically ill, liver depression must complicate their disease. This is because anyone who is chronically ill must have many unfulfilled desires. When we are ill, we can't go where we want, do what we want, eat what we want, or look the way we want. In addition, if there is chronic pain, there will also be the chronic frustration of wishing, but not being able, to get away from this pain.

The liver's coursing and discharge is intimately associated with Chinese spleen function. If the liver courses and discharges properly, then the spleen upbears the clear and the stomach downbears the turbid. Therefore, if the liver becomes depressed, almost always the spleen becomes vacuous and weak. In real life, one rarely finds one of these conditions and not the other. This is why the *Nei Jing (Inner Classic)*, the "bible" of Chinese medicine written sometime around 200 BCE says, "When the liver is diseased, first treat the spleen."

Liver depression qi stagnation can cause a wide range of health problems including FMS, chronic digestive disturbance, and emotional depression. It also plays a role in impediment conditions. Therefore, it is essential to keep the liver qi flowing freely. In following chapters, I describe a number of ways to keep the liver qi flowing freely.

2. The liver stores the blood.

This means that, when the body is at rest, the blood in the extremities returns to the liver. It is said in Chinese medicine that the liver is yin in form but yang in function. Thus the liver requires sufficient blood to keep it and its associated tissues moist and supple, cool and relaxed.

3. The liver controls the sinews.

The sinews refer mainly to the tendons and ligaments in the body. Proper function of the tendons and ligaments depends upon the nourishment of liver blood to keep them moist and supple. Chronic muscle-joint stiffness is due, in Chinese medicine, to the sinews not receiving adequate nourishment from the blood.

The heart

Although the heart is the emperor of the body-mind according to Chinese medicine, it does not play as large a role in the creation and treatment of disease as one might think. Rather than the emperor initiating the cause of disease, in Chinese medicine, mostly enduring disease eventually effects the heart. In terms of fibromyalgia, the heart is mainly involved in two ways. The first is insomnia. However, even in terms of insomnia, disturbances of the heart tend to be secondary rather than primary. By this I mean that first some other viscus or bowel becomes diseased and then the heart feels the negative effect. The basic statement of fact about the heart relating to insomnia in Chinese medicine is that:

1. The heart stores the spirit.

The spirit refers to the mind in Chinese medicine. Therefore, this statement underscores that mental function, mental clarity, and mental equilibrium are all associated with the heart. If the heart does not receive enough qi or blood or if the heart is disturbed by something, the spirit may become restless and this may produce symptoms of mental-emotional unrest, heart palpitations, insomnia, profuse dreams, etc.

According to Chinese medical theory, the heart also plays an intermediary role in the creation of the tender spots associated with FMS. The statement of fact which explains this is:

2. The heart and small intestine share a mutual interior-exterior relationship.

This means that the heart, an interior viscus, is connected to the small intestine and its paired yang, exterior channel. As we will see below in the chapter on acupuncture, the mechanism for the creation of the tender spots characteristic of fibromyalgia has to do with this heart/small intestine axis.

However, another important statement of fact about the heart which should not be overlooked is that:

3. Joy is the emotion associated with the heart.

The word joy has been interpreted by Chinese in two different ways. On the one hand, joy can mean overexcitation, in which case, excessive joy can cause problems with the heart's storing the spirit. Simply put, overexcitation may damage the heart and cause restlessness of the heart spirit, thus leading to anxiety, agitation, mood swings, and insomnia. On the other hand, joy may be seen as an antidote to the other six emotions of Chinese medicine. From this point of view, joy causes the flow of qi (and, therefore, blood) to relax and become more moderate and harmonious. If some other emotion causes the qi to become bound or move chaotically, then joy can make it relax and flow normally again. Thus anything that causes joy may help to correct and disinhibit the flow of qi and blood.

The kidneys

In Chinese medicine, the kidneys are considered to be the foundation of human life. Because the developing fetus looks like a large kidney and because the kidneys are the main organ for the storage of inherited essence, the kidneys are referred to as the prenatal root. Thus it is essential to good health and longevity to keep the kidney qi strong and kidney yin and yang in relative balance. The most important Chinese medical facts about the kidneys in terms of fibromyalgia are:

1. The kidneys are responsible for human reproduction, development, and maturation.

These are the same functions we described when we discussed the essence. This is because the essence is stored in the kidneys. Health problems related to reproduction, development, and maturation are commonly problems of kidney essence. Women's menstruation is part of reproduction and, therefore, is, at least in part, related to Chinese kidney function. Fibromyalgia is most common in women who are of menstruating age. Unfortunately, this statement also implies that the kidneys become vacuous and insufficient as we age. For instance, the *Nei Jing (Inner Classic)* says that the yin (meaning kidney yin), is half used up by 40 years of age.

2. The kidneys rule the bones and marrow.

This function includes the joints. Thus all chronic, enduring muscle-joint pain tends to involve the kidneys. Even if the disease did not start out affecting the kidneys, over time, chronic impediment conditions will inevitably involve the kidneys. In Chinese it is said, "Enduring diseases reach the kidneys."

3. The kidneys are the root of water metabolism.

The kidneys work in coordination with the lungs and spleen to insure that water fluids are spread properly throughout the body and that excess water is excreted via urination. Therefore, problems such as edema, excessive dryness, or excessive day or nighttime urination can all indicate a weakness of kidney function.

4. Kidney yin and yang are the root of the yin and yang of the entire body.

This is another way of saying that the kidneys are the foundation of our life. If either kidney yin or yang is insufficient, eventually the yin or yang of the other viscera and bowels will also become insufficient. In particular, spleen qi vacuity often evolves into kidney yang vacuity, especially in perimenopausal women, while liver blood vacuity commonly evolves into kidney yin vacuity. In terms of this latter disease mechanism, it is said, "The blood and essence share a common source," and "The liver and kidneys share a common source."

5. The low back is the mansion of the kidneys.

This means that, of all the areas of the body, the low back is the most closely related to the health of the kidneys. If the kidneys are weak, then there may be low back pain.

The channels & network vessels

Each viscus and bowel has a corresponding channel with which it is connected. In Chinese medicine, the inside of the body is made up of the viscera and bowels. The outside of the body is composed of the sinews and bones, muscles and flesh, and skin and hair. It is the channels and network vessels which connect the inside and the outside of the body. It is through these channels and network vessels that the viscera and bowels connect with their corresponding body tissues.

The channels and network vessel system is a unique feature of Chinese medicine. These channels and vessels are different from

26

the circulatory, nervous, or lymph systems. The earliest reference to these channels and vessels is in *Nei Jing (Inner Classic)*.

The channels and vessels perform two basic functions. They are the pathways by which the qi and blood circulate through the body and between the organs and tissues. Additionally, the channels connect the internal organs with the exterior part of the body. This channel and vessel system functions in the body much like the world information communication network. The channels allow the various parts of our body to cooperate and interact to maintain our lives.

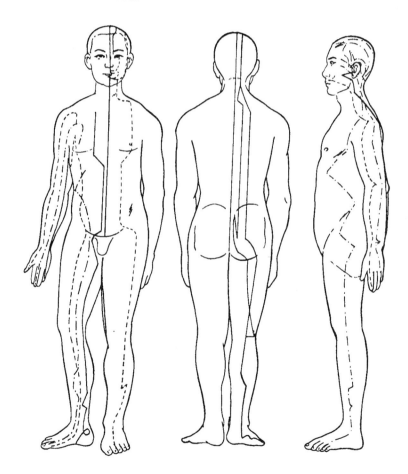

27

The channel and network vessel system is complex. There are 12 so-called regular channels, six yin and six yang, each with a specific pathway through the external body and connecting with an internal organ (see diagram). There are also extraordinary vessels, channel sinews, channel divergences, main network vessels, and ultimately countless finer and finer network vessels permeating the entire body. All of these form a closed loop or circuit that is similar to, but energetically distinct from, the circulatory system of Western medicine.

Summary

By now you should have appreciation for and a basic understanding of the holistic nature of Chinese medicine. In Chinese medicine, nothing stands alone. Every part and function in the body *co-responds* to other parts and functions in the body. The body, mind, and spirit form an integrated whole. Health is the harmonious interaction of all the various aspects that comprise the organism. Disease and pain result when there is a disruption to this fundamental harmony and balance. In Chinese medicine, the focus of treatment is the restoration of harmony. Next, let's look at the cause of pain as we explore impediment conditions according to Chinese medicine.

3
Pain According to Chinese Medicine

We have seen above that muscle-joint pain is classified as *bi* or impediment, and whenever there is impediment, there is pain. The following simple yet profound statement sums up the very essence of the Chinese medical view of pain:

> If there is free flow, there is no pain;
> If there is no free flow, there is pain.

This means that, as long as qi and blood flow freely and smoothly without hindrance or obstruction, there is no pain in the body. However, if, *due to any reason*, the flow of qi and blood is hindered, blocked, obstructed, or does not flow freely, then there will be pain. Thus, in Chinese medicine, pain is nothing other than the felt experience of lack of free flow of the qi and blood. As an extension of this, all muscle-joint pain is also nothing other than the experience of the lack of free flow of the qi and blood.

There are two main causes of the lack of free flow of the qi and blood. Either 1) something is hindering, blocking, or obstructing the smooth and uninhibited flow of qi and blood through the channels and vessels, or 2) there is insufficient qi and blood to maintain smooth and free flow. In the first case, lack of free flow is likened to a plug of hair and soap in a drainpipe. The water from the sink cannot flow freely because something is physically obstructing the pipe. In the second case, either there is insufficient qi to push the blood or insufficient blood to nourish the vessels. It is the function of the vessels to promote the flow of blood. If the vessels do not obtain sufficient blood, they cannot fulfill this function, and, therefore, the blood will cease to flow freely within them.

All pain, *no matter what its modern Western medical diagnosis*, is considered by Chinese medicine as a problem with the free flow of qi and blood. Hence, when presented with a case in which pain is an important symptom, the Chinese medicine practitioner's job is to first diagnose the reason for the non-free flow of qi and blood and, second, to provide treatment which restores that free flow.

The flow of qi and blood can become inhibited in any and every area of the body: the internal organs, the muscles, the head, the low back, and the extremities and joints. For example, when we overeat and have acute indigestion with the accompanying sensations of abdominal fullness, bloating, and distention, these symptoms are due to the stagnation of stomach qi. In this case, the stomach qi cannot move freely through the excessive amount of food and drink in the stomach. Likewise, when we bruise ourselves and blood escapes from the blood vessels and then pools, we experience a mild form of blood stagnation, technically called blood stasis in Chinese medicine. In both these cases, the stagnation is not serious. We feel better within a short time and are free of symptoms when the qi and blood resume their proper functioning and flow freely.

According to Chinese medicine, the sensations of pain due to qi stagnation or blood stasis are different. Qi stagnation causes a feeling of distention or soreness that fluctuates in intensity and location. Qi stagnation pain often occurs with strong emotional changes. Blood stasis, on the other hand, is characterized by painful swelling or stabbing sharp pain at a specific, fixed location.

It is also possible for the qi and blood flow to become inhibited because of insufficiency of the qi, blood, or both. In this case, the pain is not severe but is enduring. If due to qi and blood insufficiency, the pain is worse after rest and better after light use. This is because, during rest or immobilization, there is insufficient qi and blood to keep the qi and blood moving. Movement itself helps to pump the qi and blood through the mobilized area. Therefore, movement tends to make this type of pain better.

This is exactly what most people suffering from fibromyalgia say of their muscle-joint pain. It is worse in the morning after lying in bed and better as they move about during the day. However, all exercise and exertion does consume the qi and blood. Therefore, when pain is associated with qi and blood vacuity, light exercise improves the pain, but heavy exercise and overtaxation make it worse.

In order for a Chinese medical practitioner to diagnose and treat impediment conditions, he or she must answer the following questions:

1. Is the pain due to blockage of the qi and blood or is it due more to the insufficiency of qi and blood?
2. If the pain is due to blockage, is the pain more characteristic of qi stagnation or blood stasis?
3. What pathogenic factors are causing the qi and blood stagnation?
4. What channels or network vessels are primarily involved in the pain?
5. What internal organs are involved?

The answers to these questions directly determine the treatment the patient will receive from their Chinese medical practitioner. The basic principle of treatment in Chinese medicine is to restore balance. Therefore, the *Nei Jing (Inner Classic)* says that, if a disease is due to too much of something, that something should be drained. If it is due to too little of something, that something should be supplemented. If it is due to heat, that heat should be cooled. If it is due to cold, that cold should be warmed. If it is due to dryness, that dryness should be moistened. And if it is due to dampness, that dampness should be dried.

In Chinese medicine, two patients with the same Western medical disease may receive radically different Chinese medicine treatments because the root cause of their disease is different. This means that every patient in Chinese medicine is given an individualized treatment based on the cause and nature of their particular pattern of disharmony.

4
Impediment Conditions, Stasis & Stagnation

In the previous chapter, we saw that all pain is a reflection of a lack of free flow of either or both the qi and blood. We also saw that qi and blood may not flow freely because they either are blocked for some reason or there simply is not enough qi and blood to promote and maintain their flow. In Chinese medicine, impediment conditions not associated with a known traumatic injury are typically ascribed to blockage by either wind, cold, dampness, or heat. These are the four basic types of impediment conditions in Chinese medicine. In such cases, any one or a combination of two or more of these pathological entities may lodge in the channels and network vessels where they are not supposed to be. In that case, the qi and blood which should be freely and smoothly flowing through those channels and vessels will not be able to. It is as if there were a traffic jam. Such pathological wind, cold, dampness, or heat may either invade the body from outside or, and especially in the case of dampness and heat, may be produced internally due to any of a number of factors.

External environmental pathogens

In Chinese medicine, there are three broad categories of disease causes. These are external causes, internal causes, and neither internal nor external causes. The external causes of disease are called external environmental excesses. There are six of these external environmental excesses or pathogens. They are wind, cold, dampness, heat, dryness, and summerheat. Any of these six factors may invade the body if either of two conditions exist. First, if one or more of these factors is unusually strong or unseasonable. For instance, very cold weather in the midst of summer or very warm weather in the midst of winter may allow these "excesses" to breach the body's defensive qi and invade. Secondly, if a person's defensive qi is weaker than it should be, any of these external pathogens if present in the environment may "take advantage of this vacuity, and enter." The *Nei Jing (Inner Classic)* says, "If evils enter, there must be vacuity." This implies that evils can enter only if the defensive qi is weaker than it should be. However, there are times when the external pathogenic qi in the external environment is so strong and virulent that it can breach the stoutest defense. This is then called epidemic or pestilential qi.

Internally engendered pathogens

Although wind, cold, dampness, and heat may all potentially invade the body from outside, three of these, cold, dampness, and heat may also be produced or engendered internally. If, for any reason, there is insufficient yang qi, the body will not be as warm as it should be. The absence of heat is none other than cold. Yang qi may be damaged by overexposure to a cold environment, in which case the body exhausts itself simply maintaining its body temperature. Yang qi may be damaged by overeating uncooked, chilled foods and drinking chilled liquids, since the process of digestion is the process of turning everything that goes into the stomach into 100°F soup. Yang qi may be damaged and depleted by any loss of yin fluids, since yin fluids are the foundation or root of yang qi. Such loss of yang fluids includes bleeding, massive sweating, unrelieved vomiting, unrelieved diarrhea, or continuous, unstoppable urination. And yang qi also becomes insufficient due to the decline of visceral function in turn due to aging. If the yang qi becomes insufficient to warm the body properly, it will not propel the blood and body fluids as it should. Instead, there is constriction and retardation of flow or impediment.

Dampness may also be engendered internally due to any of several causes. Too much thinking and worry, overeating sweets, overeating damp-engendering foods, such as dairy products, wheat flour products, fruit juices, and oils and fats, and too little exercise may all damage the spleen. If the spleen is damaged and becomes weak and vacuous, then it will not move and transform body fluids properly. In that case, fluids will gather and collect and transform into dampness. Because dampness is a yin substance, it impedes the free flow of yang qi, thus resulting in *bi*. In addition, it is said in the *Nei Jing (Inner Classic)* that the spleen declines at around 35 years of age. Therefore, the spleen naturally weakens as a person ages. Consequently, one's ability to move and transform body fluids is not as good the older one gets past a certain age.

Likewise heat may be engendered internally. It does not have to invade from outside. In fact, in terms of impediment conditions, it rarely does. In order to understand how pathological heat is engendered internally resulting in impediment, one must understand that the body's healthy or correct qi (also called the righteous qi) is inherently warm in nature. If this qi backs up and accumulates for any reason, then this accumulated qi will manifest as heat. This is called transformative or depressive heat. It may be due to liver depression qi stagnation in turn transforming into depressive heat or it may be due to any other cause of blockage and obstruction. For instance, if dampness, blood, food, or phlegm gather and obstruct the free flow of yang qi, this may cause the accumulation of depressive or transformative heat. Therefore, in real life, given a sufficiency of righteous qi and either a long enough enduring or severe enough accumulation, damp impediment and even cold impediment may transform into heat impediment.

Wind

Wind is usually the primary environmental factor to invade the body. Frankly, wind here does not mean physical wind. Rather, it only refers to an unseen pathogen which affects the body mysteriously and which provokes a series of responses in the body characteristic or reminiscent of the nature of wind. Thus, a person with a windy type of pain will feel discomfort that comes and goes and moves around the body from joint to joint. Just as wind moves about the earth, the person's complaints shift throughout the body. Because wind impediment's nature is changeable or movable, this type of impediment is also called movable impediment. As mentioned above, in real life, wind as an external environmental pathogen typically combines with one of the other three. In Chinese medicine, the wind of wind impediment is primarily seen as due to external invasion.

Cold

The emblem of cold in the natural world is ice, and, therefore, when cold causes impediment, its nature and symptoms are reminiscent of ice. First, the pain of cold impediment is worsened by exposure to cold and improved by warmth or heat. Secondly, because cold is so constricting to the flow of liquids, the pain tends to be quite intense. Therefore, cold impediment is also called painful impediment. And third, just as water becomes immobile when it turns to ice, so cold impediment also tends to be fixed in location. Cold producing impediment may be due either to external invasion or internal engenderment. When one says that someone is suffering from cold impediment, all this really means is that the nature of their complaints share the characteristics of cold.

Dampness

Dampness is an accumulation of water or body fluids in the body. Because dampness is like a flood, the affected area is typically swollen and edematous. Because water tends to run downward, dampness tends to affect the lower part of the body more often than the upper part. Because water is heavy, damp impediment tends to be stationary. It does not move around from joint to joint. It is worsened by exposure to dampness and may be improved when the weather or surroundings are clear and dry. In addition, dampness tends to be lingering. Typically, damp impediment has a slow and insidious onset and then a long drawn-out course. And its pain is most often dull but persistent. Like cold above, dampness causing impediment may be due to either invasion by external dampness or internally engendered dampness, with internal engenderment being the most common in the West.

Heat

Red is the color that corresponds to fire or heat in Chinese medicine. Therefore, when there is heat impediment, the affected area is often red. The area is usually also hot to the touch, and the pain is hot or burning in nature. As discussed above, heat impediment is rarely due to external invasion of hot pathogens. Usually, heat impediment is internally engendered or is an acute exacerbation of other types of impediment.

Qi stagnation & blood stasis

As we have seen above, most cases of impediment do involve wind, cold, dampness, and/or heat. However, whether these impediments are externally invading or internally engendered, they are often complicated by other factors involving the free flow of the qi and blood. Two of the most important of these factors are qi stagnation and blood stasis.

Qi stagnation

Qi stagnation is mostly due to emotional upset, stress, and frustration. Because of inability to fulfill one's desires, the liver qi cannot spread freely. This affects the liver's job of governing coursing and discharge. Because it is the qi which moves and transforms blood, body fluids, and food, if emotional upsetment and frustration cause liver depression qi stagnation, this then will affect the flow of qi and blood of the entire body and may lead to damp accumulation, phlegm obstruction, and/or food stagnation. In terms of joint pain, we already know that, "If there is pain, there is no free flow", and previously we have taken a look

37

at the four main types of impediment conditions. Therefore, it is no wonder that liver depression qi stagnation often complicates and aggravates most, if not all, impediment complaints. On the one hand, the accumulation of dampness or heat in the body leading to impediment and, therefore, pain may be directly due to qi stagnation. On the other, if there is damp, blood, or phlegm depression in the body causing blockage and hindering free flow, this will eventually lead to or aggravate qi stagnation.

Blood stasis

Static blood, also called dead blood, malign blood, vanquished blood, and dry blood, means blood which is not moving. Rather, it obstructs the free flow of the channels and vessels the same way as silt obstructs the flow of a river or stream. Static blood may be due to traumatic injury. If traumatic injury severs the channels and vessels, the blood moves outside its vessels and then pools and accumulates. In other words, the blood can only keep flowing as long as it is inside its vessels. Once there is static blood, this yin accumulation then impedes the flow of qi and body fluids. This is why traumatic injuries are followed by swelling and inflammation. The vessels are severed and blood flows outside them. This static blood then impedes the flow of qi and body fluids. Body fluids gather and accumulate and there is edema. Qi, which is yang, accumulates and there is heat and redness or inflammation. Later, when the vessels are repaired, the qi moves the blood and body fluids through the vessels. Thus the swelling goes down, the redness and heat disappear, but the static blood which is left behind manifests as a "black and blue mark."

Because of the reciprocal relationship between the qi and blood, long-term qi stagnation will lead to blood stasis. As it is said in Chinese, "If the qi moves, the blood moves; if the qi stops, the blood stops." Therefore, *anything* which hinders and impedes the flow of qi will tend to eventually cause the complication of blood stasis. On the one hand, this means emotional upsetment and frustration. On the other, either externally invading or internally engendered impediment will also, over time, tend to become complicated by blood stasis. Further, because the blood and body fluids flow together, if one of these gathers and collects, it will hinder and obstruct the free flow of the other. Thus, over time, dampness will tend to become complicated by blood stasis, while long-term blood stasis will tend to become complicated by dampness.

Fibromyalgia pain

Now that we know something about pain in Chinese medicine and also about the concepts of impediment, stasis, and stagnation, I can say that the body pain that is characteristic of fibromyalgia is a combination of wind damp heat impediment with qi stagnation and often blood stasis as well as qi and blood vacuity failing to nourish the sinews and vessels. Although the wind component of the impediment condition may be externally invading, the dampness and heat associated with fibromyalgia are usually internally engendered—the dampness by spleen vacuity and the heat by liver depression transforming into heat. Because of long-term, enduring liver depression qi stagnation, there is both concomitant spleen vacuity and a tendency to blood stasis. Because of spleen vacuity, there is both too little qi to push the blood and too little blood to nourish the sinew vessels.

This combination of factors adequately accounts for the nature of the pain associated with fibromyalgia and with a number of other symptoms of this syndrome. The pain is generalized. Therefore, it is not due to localized traumatic injury. The pain is often severe and may be sharp or stabbing. These are characteristics of blood stasis pain. The pain may also be burning. This is heat. And the pain is worse in the morning or after prolonged inactivity. This is qi and blood vacuity pain. The muscular stiffness is due to malnourishment of the sinews as is any numbness or tingling, while the heaviness of the limbs and lack of strength suggest both qi vacuity and the presence of dampness.

5
Insomnia, Fatigue & Depression

Besides bodily pain, fibromyalgia is characterized by insomnia, fatigue, and depression. Therefore, we must also understand a little bit about the Chinese medical causes of these conditions.

Insomnia

In Chinese medicine, sleep is described as the clear yang qi sinking back into and being enfolded by yin. The rising and setting of the sun is likewise a rising and sinking of the yang qi into yin darkness. Therefore, no matter what the cause of insomnia, we know that the person's yang qi is not sinking back down into the yin and staying there quiescent as it should. In this case, either the yang qi is too strong and the yin qi is too weak, something is stirring up the yang qi abnormally, or something is blocking the yang qi so it cannot return into the yin.

In the case of fibromyalgia, the sleep disturbance that most FMS sufferers complain of is being able to initially fall asleep but then not being able to sleep restfully or waking up too early in the morning and not being able to go back to sleep. This kind of insomnia is technically referred to as matitudinal insomnia, matitudinal meaning "morning" and remember that anything past 2-3 A.M. is the early morning. In Chinese medicine, the single most common cause of matitudinal insomnia is yin vacuity. Because yin is supposed to control yang, yang qi becomes hyperactive. Because yang qi has an inherent tendency to move upward and outward, if yang qi becomes hyperactive, it typically ascends. Thus clear yang pops back up too early in the morning.

Unfortunately, women are more prone to yin vacuity than men. This is because they menstruate, gestate, and lactate. All three of these activities is either a loss or consumption of yin, blood, and body fluids. Women who are, by constitution, on the thin side and/or whose hair greys prematurely have an innate tendency towards yin vacuity. However, spleen vacuity may lead to yin vacuity in any woman since there will be less blood and fluids to transform into yin essence. Likewise, yin vacuity may be the result of any persistent, long-term pathological heat in both men and women. Heat is yang and consumes yin. Therefore, either depressive or damp heat may eventually consume and damage yin and give rise to yin vacuity heat. Other common symptoms of yin vacuity failing to control yang which then counterflows upward and becomes hyperactive include night sweats, hot flashes, and ringing in the ears. If this upwardly counterflowing heat accumulates in the heart, it may also give rise to heart palpitations and feelings of anxiousness and agitation.

In some cases of fibromyalgia, there is not actual yin vacuity but only heart blood vacuity. Nevertheless, such a heart blood vacuity may also fail to nourish and calm the heart spirit and may lead to the same kind of insomnia, restless, dream-disturbed sleep, night sweats, and palpitations.

Fatigue

Fatigue is one of the key symptoms of qi vacuity, and the main viscus responsible for engendering and transforming the qi is the spleen. Although it is said that qi vacuity of any viscus may result in fatigue, both the heart qi and lung qi come directly from the spleen. Both the heart and lung qi are made from the clear qi upborne by the spleen. The liver qi comes both from the spleen and the kidneys. However, most Chinese doctors do not even recognize the possibility of a true liver qi vacuity. And even the kidney qi rarely becomes weak all by itself. In Chinese medicine, the spleen and kidneys have a reciprocal relationship, each feeding and supporting the other. Therefore, in real-life clinical practice, either kidney qi vacuity leads to spleen qi vacuity or spleen qi vacuity leads to kidney qi vacuity. In addition, all the main Chinese medicinals which supplement and boost the qi do so by fortifying and supplementing the spleen qi. Thus, whenever fatigue is a main symptom of any disease, we know that the person's spleen qi is vacuous and weak.

Depression

Emotional depression is recognized as a clinical entity in traditional Chinese medicine just as it is in modern Western medicine. Basically, most depression and all female depression is a combination of liver depression and qi stagnation and spleen qi vacuity no matter what other disease mechanisms may also be at work. When the liver is depressed and the spleen is vacuous, Chinese doctors refer to this as a liver-spleen disharmony. Emotional depression is characterized by a reluctance and disinclination to get up, to move about, to speak, or to do anything at all. This disinclination to act is mostly a function of the liver's not coursing and discharging. If the depressed person is pushed to act against their will, they typically become angry and irritable. Anger and irritability are also liver symptoms in Chinese medicine. However, almost all emotional depression is accompanied by a deep feeling of heaviness, lack of strength, and exhaustion. These are all symptoms of spleen qi vacuity.

In real life, most people with depression have more than just liver depression and spleen vacuity. Depending on their age, bodily constitution, diet, and lifestyle, they may also have depressive heat in their stomach, heart, and/or lungs. They may have dampness, phlegm, food stagnation, and blood vacuity and/or stasis. And they may have either kidney yin or yang vacuity or both yin *and* yang vacuity. However, no matter what the other Chinese disease mechanisms they may have, at the core they will have a liver-spleen disharmony or their condition evolved out of such a disharmony over time.

It is interesting to note that the core disease mechanism of irritable bowel syndrome (IBS) is also a liver-spleen disharmony.

43

Thus, it is no mere coincidence that 40-70% of FMS sufferers also suffer from IBS. In addition, such a liver-spleen disharmony is also at the root of most women's PMS and headaches. Most women's headaches occur cyclically with the menstrual cycle. Because of liver depression combined with blood vacuity (in turn due to spleen vacuity) perimenstrually, yang qi tends to counterflow upward into the head, a bony box where it hasn't the room to move. Premenstrual breast distention and pain are also due to this same upwardly counterflowing liver qi because of blood vacuity below, while qi stagnation due to liver depression and blood stasis are the main causes of dysmenorrhea.

As it so happens, I have authored or co-authored Blue Poppy *Curing* books on insomnia, depression (with Rosa Schnyer), irritable bowel syndrome (with Jane Bean Oberski), breast disease (with Honora Lee Wolfe), PMS, and headaches. Although these books contain much of the same information included here, each of these books does go into greater detail on the causes, mechanisms, diagnosis, and treatment of each of these individual diseases. Therefore, depending on your main symptoms of fibromyalgia, you may want to look at one or more of these books as well.

6
Treatment Based on Pattern Discrimination

In Chinese medicine, treatment is given on the basis of the patient's Chinese pattern and not simply on the basis of their named disease. Fibromyalgia is a Western disease diagnosis. Likewise, impediment condition, fatigue, insomnia, and depression are all also Chinese disease diagnoses. In contradistinction, liver depression, spleen vacuity, damp heat, blood stasis, and kidney vacuity are all Chinese medical patterns. In other words, a Chinese medical pattern is different from the patient's named disease, and, in professionally practiced Chinese medicine, treatment is given primarily based on the pattern and only secondarily on the patient's disease diagnosis. Thus it is said in Chinese:

> One disease, different treatments.
> Different diseases, same treatment.

This means that two patients with the same named disease may receive very different Chinese medical treatments *if their Chinese patterns are different*, while two patients with different named diseases may receive the same treatment *if their Chinese patterns are the same*. Because Chinese medicine treatments are based upon identifying an individual's unique pattern, Chinese medicine causes no side effects or other medically induced problems.

A person's Chinese pattern takes into account all the signs and symptoms of the disease plus all the patient's other, seemingly unrelated, signs and symptoms *and* the Chinese description of the cause of their condition. Therefore, all the person's symptoms are noteworthy, not just the ones that are specific to the major complaint. In fact, the Chinese medicine practitioner gathers so much information, the patient may not see the relevance of it all. A typical first interview takes from 45 minutes to an hour in order to gather all the necessary information for a comprehensive assessment. Certainly the Chinese medicine practitioner takes much more time to ask questions about all aspects of the person's life in contrast to the 15 minute exam common with the typical Western MD.

As we have seen in the previous chapters, impediment conditions causing muscle-joint pain are due to a lack of free flow of the qi and/or blood due to impediment by wind, cold, dampness or heat as well as qi stagnation, blood stasis, qi and blood vacuity, and vacuities of the spleen and kidneys. Hence, there are a number of different factors accounting for any given person's individualized signs and symptoms of fibromylagia. This means that, in Chinese medicine, each patient with fibromyalgia syndrome will receive their own, uniquely tailored treatment plan in turn based on their unique pattern of disharmony. It is only by obtaining *all* the person's signs and symptoms that the practitioner can begin to identify all the factors that contribute to this individual's FMS.

How Chinese medicine patterns are determined

How does a Chinese medical practitioner determine the pattern of disharmony that is causing an individual's fibromyalgia? First, the practitioner must have a good understanding of the theories of Chinese medicine. This includes an in-depth knowledge of qi and blood, viscera and bowels, channels and network vessels, and yin and yang and how these interconnect and interact. Secondly, the practitioner must understand how illness develops and how injury affects the body. Third, the patterns of illness that develop due to external invasion, internal damage, or traumatic injury must be understood and discriminated. Keeping all of this theoretical information in mind, the practitioner then obtains information from the patient.

The four examinations

For over 2000 years, Chinese medical practitioners have used what are called the four examinations for obtaining information about a patient's condition. These four examinations are 1) looking, 2) listening/smelling, 3) asking, and 4) touching.

1. Looking

Looking focuses on what the practitioner can see with their unaided eyes (except for normal corrective lenses). Everything about the patient that can be observed can be useful. This includes their facial expression, the brightness of their eyes, their facial complexion, bodily constitution, posture and manner of movement, inspection of the affected area, and examination of the tongue and its coating.

Tongue diagnosis is a highly developed skill in Chinese medicine and a major source of information about a patient's condition. Both the tongue itself and its coating are indicators of the person's condition. For example, a thick, greasy, yellow tongue coating indicates the presence of damp heat, while a shiny, red tongue without a coating indicates a yin vacuity.

2. Listening & smelling

Listening and smelling are the second method of examination in Chinese medicine. The character in the Chinese language for this examination means both listening *and* smelling as a single concept. (This underscores that Chinese medicine divides up the pie of reality in a very different way than how we do in English.) The practitioner listens to the patient's breathing, the quality of their voice, or other sounds, such as a cough. For example, a person with a weak voice who coughs when active may have weak qi. Body odors and the smells of any excretions also give the practitioner useful information about the patient's pattern.

3. Questioning

Questioning the patient is the third method of examination. These questions include when and how the problem happened, how long it has gone on, what treatment has already been given and with what results, general medical history, sensations of cold and heat, location and quality of pain, descriptions of urination and bowel movements, sleep patterns, perspiration, headaches, dizziness, appetite, thirst, digestive disturbances, energy level, gynecological problems, and more. Because the sensations of pain due to stagnation of qi and blood differ as do the pain and aching due to the various types of *bi*, the patient's description of the pain is critical in determining what type of *bi* or what type of pattern exists.

4. Palpation

Palpation or touch is the last method of examination. The most important aspect of this method, at least in terms of assessing viscera and bowel function and basic quantities and qualities of qi and blood flow, is taking the pulse. Together with the information gained from examining the tongue, taking the pulse is central to Chinese medical diagnosis. Chinese pulse diagnosis requires great skill and sensitivity. The pulse taken at the wrist provides information about the basic state of the person's qi and blood, yin and yang, viscera and bowels, and pathogenic factors. There are 28 different standard pulse qualities described in the classical literature. For example, people in pain who have a lot of qi and blood typically have a pulse which is tight "like a taut rope", while people in pain with less qi and blood typically have a pulse which is wiry "like the string of a zither."

However, the Chinese practitioner not only palpates the pulse but will also palpate the body in any areas the patient says are painful. The 18 painful points of fibromyalgia are all standard acupuncture points or are located along the course of the 12 regular channels. By knowing which of these 18 are painful, one immediately knows in which channels the qi and blood is not flowing freely. This is useful both for the acupuncture treatment of these channels and also for understanding the underlying viscera and bowel dysfunction associated with this lack of free flow in the channels and vessels.

By gathering information through the four examinations and by comparing the patient's signs and symptoms with the condition of the tongue and pulse, the patient's pattern is understood and named. The name of the pattern describes an inherent state of imbalance. For instance, kidney yin insufficiency means that kidney yin is too weak. Therefore, the next step is creating a treatment plan which will correct the imbalance implied in the name of the pattern. If there is kidney yin vacuity, the kidneys should be supplemented and yin should be nourished or enriched. Hence treatment techniques are applied to bring about this result, the return to balance and, therefore, health.

7
The Pattern Discrimination of Fibromyalgia

Although each patient with the Western diagnosis of fibromyalgia will have their own uniquely tailored Chinese pattern discrimination, based on both the published Chinese medical literature on fibromyalgia and my more than 20 years of clinical experience, there are certain patterns that are at the core of most people's FMS. These patterns are spleen qi and liver blood-kidney yin vacuity (usually abbreviated to simply qi and yin vacuity) with wind damp heat impediment complicated by liver depression qi stagnation and possibly by blood stasis. Then, depending on the patient's sex, age, diet, lifestyle, and constitution, they may have any of a number of other complicating patterns that are evolutions or off-shoots of these main or core patterns. If one understands these main and subsidiary patterns, one can understand why any particular patient has the complex constellation of signs and symptoms they do.

Below are the signs, symptoms, and treatment principles for each of the main patterns of FMS. They are presented as discreet, individual patterns with their textbook signs and symptoms. However, in real life, the mechanisms associated with these patterns modify each other's symptoms when they occur simultaneously. Therefore, unlike most standard Chinese medical textbooks, I have also tried to give some indications of these real-life modifications. While all these core patterns tend to occur at the same time, their proportions or preponderances shift from individual to individual and from time to time. That is why there is no "one size fits all" treatment for fibromyalgia. In any case, hopefully you will be able to see yourself in the patterns presented below. If you can, I'm sure you will be able to find numerous hints and suggestions in the following chapters to help get you back on the road to pain-free, vibrant good health and abundant energy.

Spleen qi vacuity

Main symptoms: Fatigue, loss of strength in the extremities, loose stools or diarrhea, increased number of bowel movements, especially after eating, reduced appetite, stomach and epigastric distention and fullness after eating, superficial edema, *i.e.*, swelling or puffiness, cold hands and feet, easy bruising, heavy menstruation or abnormal uterine bleeding, dizziness upon standing up, a pale facial complexion, a fat tongue with thin, white fur, and a fine, weak pulse

Treatment principles: Fortify the spleen and supplement the qi

Because adipose tissue is considered dampness and phlegm in Chinese medicine and "the spleen is the root of phlegm engenderment," many patients with spleen vacuity tend to be overweight even though obesity is not considered, *per se*, a symptom of spleen vacuity.

Liver depression qi stagnation

Main symptoms: Irritability, mental-emotional depression, constipation with thin, ribbon-like or small round stools or diarrhea alternating with constipation, burping and belching, chest, rib-side and abdominal distention or pain, premenstrual breast distention and pain, painful menstruation, a normal or slightly dark tongue with thin, white fur, and a bowstring[1] pulse

---

[1] There are 28 main pulse types in Chinese medicine, the bowstring pulse being one of these. It feels like its name implies—like a taut violin or bowstring.

Treatment principles: Course the liver and rectify the qi

Damp heat

Main symptoms: Loose stools or diarrhea, possibly dark, green-colored stools or light, yellow, mustard-colored stools, a burning or acid feeling around the anus with or after defecation, foul-smelling stools, hot, possibly red, possibly swollen, painful limbs, red, hot, swollen, wet, or weeping skin lesions, hot, frequent, burning, and/or painful urination, red, hot, swollen, wet or weeping external genitalia, thick white, curdy or creamy yellow abnormal vaginal discharge, yellow-green nasal mucus, slimy, yellow tongue fur, and a slippery, rapid pulse

Treatment principles: Clear heat and eliminate dampness

Damp heat manifests somewhat differently depending in which part of the body it is lodged. Areas of the body commonly affected by damp heat include the reproductive tract and external genitalia, the urinary tract, the digestive tract, the lower limbs, and the skin. Patients with damp heat typically exhibit that damp heat in two or more of these areas but rarely in all of them at the same time. It is common for damp heat to migrate from system to system within the body, sometimes manifesting as urinary tract damp heat, other times as gastrointestinal damp heat, and yet other times as dermatological damp heat. When damp heat causes impediment pain, this is also often called wind damp heat impediment. Because the heat of damp heat does tend to waft upwards, damp heat below can also give rise to signs and symptoms of dry heat above, such as heat in the heart or dry mouth and throat and chapped lips.

Blood vacuity

Main symptoms: Pale nails, pale lips, a pale, white or sallow, yellow facial complexion, brittle nails, constipation with dry stools, poor sleep, dry skin or hair, muscular stiffness, tension, or cramps, numbness and/or tingling in the extremities, itching, blurred vision, night blindness, dizziness, heart palpitations, anxiety, poor memory, a pale tongue with dryish fur, and a fine pulse

Treatment principles: Nourish and supplement the blood

The signs and symptoms of blood vacuity vary depending on which viscera are affected. Pain, numbness, brittle nails, and vision problems are related to the liver. Constipation in this pattern is due to blood vacuity leading to fluid dryness in the large intestine. While heart blood vacuity is characterized by palpitations, poor memory, anxiety and disturbed sleep. The remainder of the symptoms are characteristic of blood vacuity in general.

Kidney yin vacuity/vacuity heat

Main symptoms: Low back pain and knee soreness, nighttime urination, frequent but scanty, darkish urination, dizziness, tinnitus, early morning insomnia, night sweats, hot flashes, heat in the palms and soles of the feet, a red tongue with no or scanty fur, and a fine, rapid, or floating, surging, rapid pulse

Treatment principles: Supplement the kidneys, enrich yin, and clear vacuity heat

Blood stasis

Main symptoms: Fixed, sharp, stabbing and/or severe pain which is commonly worse in the evening and at night, engorged visible blood vessels, from large varicosities to spider nevi and cherry hemangiomas, engorged and distended sublingual veins, painful menstruation, blood clots in the menstruate, blood clots in any visible bleeding, a dark, sooty facial complexion, liver or age spots, a dark, possibly purplish tongue or static spots or black and blue marks on the tongue, and a bowstring, choppy, deep, slow, and/or irregular pulse

Treatment principles: Quicken the blood and dispel stasis

Blood stasis complicates most chronic, enduring diseases.

The following patterns commonly complicate the above core patterns of FMS. Their existence is more variable than those already discussed. While most people have varying proportions of the above patterns, only some people also display the following patterns.

Kidney yang vacuity

Main symptoms: Possible daybreak diarrhea (*i.e.*, diarrhea very early in the morning), weakness or soreness in the low back or knees, decreased libido, frequent urination, waking at night to urinate, cold lower half of the body and especially the feet, a pale tongue with a thin, white coating and a deep, slow and forceless pulse

Treatment principles: Supplement the kidneys and invigorate yang

This pattern is a typical complication of FMS in perimenopausal women. It most commonly shows up after 40 years of age. Since it complicates already existing liver depression qi stagnation and spleen qi vacuity it will not be seen clinically in the textbook form described above. Typically, as few as two or three of the symptoms of kidney yang vacuity will be present along with the symptoms of the main patterns. In particular, the tongue and pulse will tend to reflect the main patterns. Therefore, the tongue or at least its tip may actually be red and the pulse may be floating and fast as opposed to the textbook form of slow and deep. For me, if a woman is more than 40 years of age and has three out of the following four key symptoms, I believe she has kidney yang vacuity no matter what other patterns are also presenting: low back pain, nocturia, cold feet, and/or decreased sexual desire.

Defensive qi not securing

Main symptoms: Easy perspiration, easy invasion by external evils, possible shortness of breath

Treatment principles: Supplement the qi and secure the exterior

This pattern is actually only a complication of spleen qi vacuity. The lungs govern the defensive qi which guards the exterior of the body from invasion by external evils. If the spleen qi is vacuous and weak, so will be the lung qi. If the lung qi is vacuous and weak, so will be the defensive qi. In that case, the person will not only catch flus and colds easily, they are also prone to allergies. In other words, they are easily invaded by unseen airborne pathogens that do not cause any problems to those with normally healthy defensive qi. This pattern is present in all persons with respiratory allergies, such as hayfever and asthma, even though they may not have the easy perspiration and shortness of breath the Chinese textbooks always mention.

Phlegm nodulation

Main symptoms: Swollen lymph nodes, fibrocystic lumps in the breast, other hard, round, subcutaneous lumps and bumps

Treatment principles: Transform phlegm and scatter nodulation

As mentioned previously, the spleen is the root of phlegm engenderment. If the spleen is vacuous and weak, it may fail to move and transport body fluids which then gather and collect, transforming into pathological dampness. If dampness endures, and especially if it is further worked on by either cold or heat, it may congeal into phlegm. People who catch recurrent infections and have sore throats often have swollen glands which are considered to be phlegm nodulations in Chinese medicine. Likewise, the lumps of fibrocystic breast disease are also considered phlegm nodulations. Although the nasal discharge of allergic rhinitis and the phlegm in asthma are not nodulations, they are signs of abnormally profuse phlegm.

Since it is not always easy to see oneself, the best way to determine your exact mix of Chinese patterns and their complications is to seek a professional diagnosis by a local practitioner of Chinese medicine. Also please remember that, unlike your Western disease diagnosis, your Chinese pattern discrimination may change from week to week due to your menstrual cycle, the phases of the moon, the weather outside, and your diet, lifestyle, and mood. This is why professional practitioners of Chinese medicine like to see or at least talk to their patients once a week during active treatment phases.

8
How This System Works in Real Life

Hannah from Chapter 1 has decided to see a professional practitioner of Chinese medicine. When she arrived at this practitioner's office, they had her fill out a lengthy intake form asking her both about her current symptoms and her medical history. When she went into the practitioner's office, they asked her even more questions about every aspect of her body's functioning. Then the practitioner had Hannah stick out her tongue several times. And finally, the practitioner asked Hannah to put both wrists palm up on a small cushion and felt the pulses in both her wrists. During all of this, the practitioner was taking copious notes. After writing down the pulse findings, the practitioner went over everything in front of them and asked a few more questions. Finally the practitioner told Hannah her Chinese pattern discrimination. Hannah was exhibiting a (spleen) qi and (liver blood-kidney) yin vacuity with damp heat, liver depression, and blood stasis.

How did the practitioner know all this?

Right away, the practitioner knew that Hannah was exhibiting spleen qi vacuity because of her extreme exhaustion and fatigue. They also took into account the facts that she was a female, that she was 40 years of age, and that she was slightly overweight. Spleen qi vacuity was then confirmed by the facts that her fatigue was worse after eating and she developed abdominal distention after meals. Hannah had also said yes to lack of strength and dizziness when she stood up as well as easy bruising, all common spleen qi vacuity signs and symptoms.

Spleen qi vacuity was also confirmed by her swollen, enlarged tongue and a pulse which was fine, floating, and forceless in the middle position on her right hand.

The practitioner suspected Hannah was exhibiting a liver blood-kidney yin vacuity because of her matitudinal insomnia and muscular stiffness. In addition, Hannah was prematurely grey. Liver blood-kidney yin vacuity was confirmed by the facts that her pulse was very fine overall on the left wrist and her tongue was pale but its tip was abnormally red. To further confirm a liver blood vacuity, the practitioner had ascertained that Hannah did not see very well at night and her fingernails were dry and brittle. To further confirm the kidney yin vacuity, the practitioner had ascertained that Hannah had low back pain and had to get up at night to urinate. However, when she did so, her urine was scanty and dark yellow in color.

The damp heat was evidenced by the hot, heavy feelings Hannah had in all the joints which were sore and the fact that this muscular aching and soreness was worse when the weather was damp and hot. It was also evidenced by the slightly yellow, slimy coating on the back of Hannah's tongue, the slippery quality of the pulse in the proximal position on the right wrist, her sometimes dark and sometimes bright yellow stools, and the burning feeling she had around her anus after defecation. It was further confirmed by the fact that Hannah had a history of urinary tract infections that had been treated by antibiotics and sometimes had "yeasty" or curdy vaginal discharge which was aggravated by eating sugar and sweets.

The fact that Hannah was depressed and that her PMS had worsened immediately made the practitioner suspect liver depression qi stagnation. This was confirmed by the abdominal cramping before bowel movements, her irritability, and a worsening of all her symptoms when under emotional stress. Besides that, her pulses were also definitely bowstring, the pulse of the liver. Given all that was going wrong for Hannah in her body, the practitioner would have been surprised if there hadn't been plenty of signs and symptoms of liver depression.

And finally, the fact that Hannah had blood stasis was suggested by the severe, sharp, fixed nature of some of Hannah's body pain and was further borne out by her severe menstrual cramps, the clots in her menstruate, and the pronounced varicosities behind her left knee.

What to do about all of this?

Although Hannah has a number of Chinese patterns presenting simultaneously, this seeming complexity really does not present any particular problem to the Chinese doctor. Having determined Hannah's overall pattern, the Chinese medical practitioner next states the treatment principles necessary to correct the imbalances implied in the names of Hannah's patterns. Thus the next thing the Chinese doctor does is write down the following principles:

Fortify the spleen and boost the qi, nourish the blood and enrich yin, clear heat and eliminate dampness, course the liver and rectify the qi, quicken the blood and free the flow of the network vessels

Knowing that these are the treatment principles that will restore balance to Hannah's system, anything that promotes these principles will be good for Hannah, and anything that goes against these principles will be bad for Hannah. In terms of professional therapies, the two main professional modalities used by Chinese doctors are Chinese herbal medicine and acupuncture. There are Chinese medicinal herbs whose functions are to fortify the spleen and boost the qi. There are other Chinese herbs which nourish the blood and enrich yin. Yet other Chinese herbs clear heat and eliminate dampness, course the liver and rectify the qi, or quicken the blood and free the flow of the network vessels. Therefore, the Chinese doctor will write a prescription for Chinese herbs that cover all these bases. Likewise, there are acupuncture points which also perform these

61

various functions. Here in the West, most Chinese medical practitioners practice both herbal medicine and acupuncture, so Hannah will probably receive treatment with both of these modalities.

In addition, the Chinese medical practitioner will pay careful attention to Hannah's diet. Because spleen qi vacuity plays such an important part in fibromyalgia and because the spleen is so easily damaged by eating the wrong things, the right diet is the foundation of its treatment. (We will discuss the correct diet for most fibromyalgia sufferers in a subsequent chapter.) However, Hannah's practitioner will also discuss the importance of proper exercise and rest and also of daily deep relaxation. By taking her Chinese herbs and receiving some acupuncture treatments as well as following her practitioner's advice regarding diet, exercise, relaxation, and lifestyle, Hannah should be well on her way to recovery by the end of three months.

What if Hannah had had other symptoms?

If Hannah had had other symptoms than the ones we have discussed above, then her Chinese pattern or combination of patterns would be slightly different or at least the order of their importance would be different. For instance, if Hannah had wet eczema as well as frequent, burning urination at the time of her examination, damp heat might have been moved to the head of the list. If Hannah had complained of hayfever and/or asthma, phlegm dampness would have been added to her list of other patterns, perhaps after liver depression and before blood stasis. If Hannah had said that, in addition to everything else, she had cold feet and markedly decreased libido, then we would've added kidney yang vacuity after liver blood-kidney yin vacuity or we simply might have said she had a dual kidney yin and yang vacuity. In other words, if a person's symptom-sign complex changes in any way, then their Chinese pattern discrimination does also, and professional Chinese medical care is primarily predicated upon each patient's pattern.

9
Chinese Herbal Medicine & Fibromyalgia

As we have seen from Hannah's case above, there is no one Chinese "fibromylagia herb" or even a single "fibromyalgia formula." Chinese medicinals are individually prescribed based on a person's pattern discrimination, not on a disease diagnosis like FMS. The pattern discrimination is very important because if, for example, a person has FMS and most of her symptoms are due to liver depression, then too many qi supplements or too high a dose of them will make the person feel worse, not better. Since this person's qi is depressed, adding more qi to what is already not flowing freely only adds to this depression and may worsen the symptoms that are due to it, such as abdominal pain, constipation, or irritability.

In addition, because most people with FMS present with more than one Chinese pattern and disease mechanism, professional Chinese medicine never treats those with FMS with herbal "singles." In Western herbalism, singles mean the prescription of a single herb all by itself. Chinese herbal medicine is based on rebalancing patterns, and patterns in real-life patients almost always have more than a single element. Therefore, Chinese doctors almost always prescribe herbs in multi-ingredient formulas. Such formulas may have anywhere from six to eighteen or more ingredients. When a Chinese doctor reads a prescription by another Chinese doctor, they can tell you not only what the patient's pattern discrimination is but also their probable signs and symptoms. In other words, the Chinese doctor does not just combine several medicinals which are all reputed to be "good for FMS." Rather, they carefully craft a formula whose ingredients are meant to rebalance every aspect of the patient's body–mind.

Getting your own individualized prescription

In China, it takes not less than four years of full-time college education to learn how to do a professional Chinese pattern discrimination and then write an herbal formula based on that pattern discrimination, most lay people cannot realistically write their own Chinese herbal prescriptions. It should also be remembered that Chinese herbs are not effective and safe because they are either Chinese or herbal. In fact, approximately 20% of the common Chinese materia medica did not originate in China, and not all Chinese herbs are completely safe. They are only safe when prescribed according to a correct pattern discrimination, in the right dose, and for the right amount of time. After all, if an herb is strong enough to heal an imbalance, it is also strong enough to create an imbalance if overdosed or misprescribed. Therefore, I strongly recommend that those who wish to experience the many benefits of Chinese herbal medicine see a qualified professional practitioner who can do a professional pattern discrimination and write an individualized prescription. Towards the end of this book, I will give suggestions on how to find such a practitioner.

Experimenting with Chinese patent medicines

In reality, qualified professional practitioners of Chinese medicine are not yet found in every North American and European community. In addition, some people may want to try to heal their FMS as much on their own as possible. More and more health food stores are stocking a variety of ready-made Chinese formulas in pill and powder form. These ready-made, over-the-counter Chinese medicines are often referred to as Chinese patent medicines. Although my best recommendation is for people to seek Chinese herbal treatment from professional practitioners, below are some suggestions of how one might experiment with Chinese patent medicines to treat FMS.

In Chapter 7, I have given the signs and symptoms of the core patterns associated with most cases of FMS. These are:

1. Spleen qi vacuity
2. Liver blood-kidney yin vacuity
3. Damp heat
4. Liver depression qi stagnation
5. Blood stasis

The first step in choosing a formula is to identify the main pattern or patterns causing your FMS. After you have done that, you can consider trying one or more of the following Chinese patent remedies. Because FMS includes a number of patterns and so many different symptoms, you will most likely have to use more than one of these medicines at the same time in order to cover all your patterns.

Dang Gui Nian Tong Tang

The name of this formula translates as "Dang Gui Assuage Pain Decoction." Dang Gui is the Chinese name of one of the main ingredients in this formula. This formula was created by Li Dong-yuan at the time of Genghis Khan. Li was a master of composing complex formulas for people with muscle joint pain, spleen vacuity, liver depression, and some kind of pathological heat. The ingredients in this formula are:

Radix Angelicae Sinensis (*Dang Gui*)
Radix Codonopsitis Pilosulae (*Dang Shen*)
Rhizoma Atractylodis Macrocephalae (*Bai Zhu*)
Rhizoma Atractylodis (*Cang Zhu*)
Sclerotium Polypori Umbellati (*Zhu Ling*)
Rhizoma Alismatis (*Ze Xie*)
Rhizoma Anemarrhenae Aspheloidis (*Zhi Mu*)
Radix Scutellariae Baicalensis (*Huang Qin*)
Herba Artemisiae Capillaris (*Yin Chen Hao*)
Radix Sophorae Flavescentis (*Ku Shen*)
Radix Puerariae (*Ge Gen*)

Radix Et Rhizoma Notopterygii (*Qiang Huo*)
Radix Ledebouriellae Divaricatae (*Fang Feng*)
Rhizoma Cimicifugae (*Sheng Ma*)
Radix Glycyrrhizae (*Gan Cao*)

This formula is indicated for the treatment of wind damp heat impediment with spleen qi vacuity, liver blood-kidney yin vacuity, liver depression, and blood stasis, the exact same set of core patterns so commonly seen in fibromyalgia patients. However, in the case of this formula, liver blood and kidney yin vacuities are relatively minor as is the blood stasis. The main emphasis in this formula is on treating damp heat impediment and supplementing the spleen.

Within this formula, Ginseng, Atractylodes Macrocephala, and Atractylodes (a.k.a. Atractylis) fortify the spleen, supplement the qi, and dry dampness. Polyporus and Alisma aid in the elimination of dampness by seeping or percolating it. This means they promote urination. Dang Gui both nourishes and quickens the blood. Scutellaria, Artemisia Capillaris, and Sophora clear heat and eliminate dampness. Artemisia Capillaris has some ability to also course the liver and rectify the qi. Cimicifuga and Pueraria both upbear clear yang and therefore also rectify the qi and resolve depression. Pueraria also works with Notopterygium and Ledebouriella to dispel wind damp and free the flow of impediment. Further, Pueraria nourishes stomach yin, thus protecting fluids from damage due to the use of acrid, "windy," drying medicinals. Anemarrhena nourishes the kidneys and clears vacuity heat, while Licorice clears heat and harmonizes the other medicinals while protecting the stomach.

If there is more pronounced blood vacuity, yin vacuity, or blood stasis, this formula can be combined with one of the others discussed below which address these patterns more forcefully. This formula is currently available as a desiccated extract in both powder and capsule forms.

Caution: If one tries this formula or any of the following formulas and experiences *any side effects*, please stop its use immediately and seek the guidance of a qualified professional practitioner of Chinese herbal medicine.

Xiao Feng San Wan

This formula is also for the treatment of damp heat impediment body pain. It was created by Chen Shi-gong in the late 1500s or early 1600s. Therefore, it has proven its clinical efficacy over 400 years. Its name means "Disperse Wind Powder Pills."[1] Its ingredients include:

Radix Ledebouriellae Divaricatae (*Fang Feng*)
Radix Sophorae Flavescentis (*Ku Shen*)
Gypsum Fibrosum (*Shi Gao*)
uncooked Radix Rehmanniae (*Sheng Di*)
Herba Seu Flos Schizonepetae Tenuifoliae (*Jing Jie*)
Periostracum Cicadae (*Chan Tui*)
Fructus Arctii Lappae (*Niu Bang Zi*)
black Semen Sesami Indici (*Hei Zhi Ma*)
Rhizoma Anemarrhenae Aspheloidis (*Zhi Mu*)
Radix Angelicae Sinensis (*Dang Gui*)
Rhizoma Atractylodis (*Cang Zhu*)
Caulis Akebiae (*Mu Tong*)
Radix Glycyrrhizae (*Gan Cao*)

This formula not only treats wind damp heat impediment pain, it also treats damp heat that may be causing skin conditions characterized by redness, swelling, heat, wetness or oozing, and itching. It nourishes the blood and enriches kidney yin. It also quickens and frees the flow of the network vessels. Its ingredients also suggest it might be helpful for cases of FMS

---

[1] Because many of the medicines in this section were originally designed as powders or decoctions, they often have the words "powder" or "decoction" in their name followed by the word "pill." this suggests that these formulas have only recently become available in pill form.

accompanied by restless leg syndrome as well as by numbness and tingling. However, it does *not* treat spleen vacuity.

Within this formula, Ledebouriella, Schizonepeta, Arctium, and Atractylis are all wind damp impediment medicinals. In addition, Atractylis also dries dampness. Therefore, it helps Akebia eliminate dampness. Akebia disinhibits urination and seeps dampness. There are four ingredients in this formula which clear heat. Sophora clears heat and eliminates dampness, Anemarrhena clears vacuity heat and enriches kidney yin, uncooked Rehmannia clears heat and cools and moistens the blood, and Gypsum clears heat and drains fire. Uncooked Rehmannia also helps Dang Gui both nourish and quicken the blood. Likewise, black Sesame Seeds nourish the blood and moisten dryness, thus aiding the nourishment of the sinews and skin. Licorice harmonizes all the rest of the medicinals in this formula and helps prevent any of them from damaging the spleen and stomach.

Because almost all cases of fibromyalgia also include spleen qi vacuity and liver depression, this formula should be combined with *Xiang Sha Liu Jun Zi Wan* discussed below to supplement the spleen and boost the qi, course the liver and rectify the qi. This formula can also be combined with other Chinese ready-made medicines if there is more pronounced liver depression, yin or yang vacuities, or blood stasis. It is currently available in pill and powdered extract forms.

Si Miao San Wan

This formula was created by Zhang Bing-cheng sometime around 1904. However, it is based on another formula created by Yu Tian-min in 1515 to which Zhang only added one ingredient. It is another famous Chinese herbal formula for the treatment of wind damp heat impediment pain. Its name means "Four Miracles Powder Pills," and its ingredients are:

Semen Coicis Lachryma-jobi (*Yi Yi Ren*)
Radix Achyranthis Bidentatae (*Niu Xi*)

Rhizoma Atractylodis (*Cang Zhu*)
Cortex Phellodendri (*Huang Bai*)

This formula is indicated for wind damp heat impediment which is primarily effecting the lower limbs and may be accompanied by swelling and puffiness of the lower legs or damp hot skin lesions on the lower half of the body. It supplements the spleen and kidneys only minimally (some might even say not at all). Coix or Job's Tears Barley seeps dampness and does fortify the spleen somewhat. Achyranthes nourishes the liver and kidneys, strengthens the sinews and the bones, and also leads the blood downward and quickens the blood in the lower half of the body. Atractylis dries dampness and also treats wind damp impediment pain, while Phellodendron clears heat and eliminates dampness.

Because fibromylagia is so much more complicated than just wind damp heat impediment pain, this formula will have to be combined with one or more other formulas to supplement the spleen and boost the qi, course the liver and resolve depression, supplement the liver and kidneys, and quicken the blood and dispel stasis. Nevertheless, when combined with the appropriate other formulas, it can be very useful in treating the body pain of fibromyalgia. Although originally a powder, this medicine now comes in pills and powdered extract form.

Huo Luo Xiao Ling Dan Wan

The name of this Chinese herbal formula translates as "Fantastically Effective Network Vessel Quickening Elixir Pills." It was created by Zhang Xi-chun sometime during the late Nineteenth century and definitely before 1934. It is for the treatment of body pain due to blood stasis in the network vessels. It is comprised of:

Radix Angelicae Sinensis (*Dang Gui*)
Resina Olibani (*Ru Xiang*)
Resina Myrrhae (*Mo Yao*)
Radix Salviae Miltiorrhizae (*Dan Shen*)

Dang Gui both nourishes and quickens the blood; so does Salvia. However, Dang Gui primarily nourishes the blood and only secondarily quickens it, while Salvia primarily quickens the blood and only secondarily nourishes it. Olibanum or Frankincense and Myrrh are a commonly used combination in Chinese herbal medicine in order to free the flow of the network vessels and stop pain. Therefore, this handy patent medicine can be combined with other Chinese ready-made medicines when there is more significant blood stasis. For instance, it might be combined with either *Dang Gui Nian Tong Tang* or *Si Miao San Wan* discussed above if blood stasis were more severe and apparent.

Qing Gu San Wan

The Chinese word *qing* means to "clear" as in clearing heat. *Gu* means bones, *san* means powder and/or to scatter, and *wan* means "pills". Therefore, the whole name of this formula means "Clear the Bones Powder Pills." It was created by Wang Ken-tang in the late 1500s or very early 1600s and is indicated for yin vacuity/vacuity heat with a hot, steaming feeling deep in the bones as if one's bones were steaming. Its ingredients are:

Radix Stellariae Dichotomae (*Yin Chai Hu*)
Rhizoma Anemarrhenae Aspheloidis (*Zhi Mu*)
Rhizoma Picrorrhizae (*Hu Huang Lian*)
Cortex Radicis Lycii Chinensis (*Di Gu Pi*)
Herba Artemisiae Apiaceae (*Qing Hao*)
Radix Gentianae Macrophyllae (*Qin Jiao*)
Carapax Amydae Sinensis (*Bie Jia*)
Radix Glycyrrhizae (*Gan Cao*)

This formula can be combined with other formulas for fibromyalgia when yin vacuity/vacuity heat is more pronounced, such as in the case of night sweats and low-grade fever. Stellaria and Cortex Lycii both clear vacuity heat. So does Anemarrhena, Artemisia Apiacea, and Gentiana. However, Anemarrhena also enriches kidney yin, while Artemisia Apiacea also clears summerheat. Summerheat is a kind of damp heat, usually found in tandem with spleen qi vacuity. And Gentiana also treats wind damp impediment pain. Picrorrhiza clears heat and eliminates dampness. Carapax Amydae quickens the blood in the network vessels, enriches yin, downbears upwardly counterflowing yang, and does have some ability to also clear heat and eliminate dampness. And Licorice harmonizes all the rest of the medicinals in the formula.

This formula comes in pill form. It can be added to other ready-made Chinese medicines which supplement the spleen and course the liver when yin vacuity with vacuity heat is pronounced.

Ba Zheng San Wan

The name of this formula means "Eight (Ingredients) Correcting Powder Pills." It is for the treatment of damp heat in the bladder causing hot, burning, frequent, painful, stuttering or choppy urination. It was first recorded in the Chinese medical literature around the time of William the Conqueror or 1066 CE. Its ingredients are:

Caulis Akebiae (*Mu Tong*)
Talcum (*Hua Shi*)
Semen Plantaginis (*Che Qian Zi*)
Herba Dianthi (*Qu Mai*)
Herba Polygoni Avicularis (*Bian Xu*)
Fructus Gardeniae Jasminoidis (*Zhi Zi*)
Radix Et Rhizoma Rhei (*Da Huang*)
Herba Lysimachiae (*Jin Qian Cao*)
Radix Glycyrrhizae (*Gan Cao*)

Akebia, Talcum, Plantago, Dianthus, and Polygonum Avicularis all disinhibit urination and seep dampness. Gardenia and Lysimachia both clear heat and eliminate dampness. And Licorice harmonizes all the other medicinals in this medicine. It is available in pill and powdered extract form and can be combined with other Chinese ready-made medicines when damp heat in the bladder is causing urinary problems.

71

Tong Xie Yao Fang

Tong Xie Yao Fang means "Painful Diarrhea Essential Formula." Happily, this famous formula for spleen vacuity and liver depression with abdominal cramping and diarrhea is now available in pill form as well as a desiccated extract powder. This is the single most commonly prescribed Chinese medicinal formula for irritable bowel syndrome or IBS. Therefore, it can be combined with other Chinese ready-made medicines when a liver-spleen disharmony is causing abdominal cramping and diarrhea. This formula was created by Zhang Jie-bin in the early 1600s. Its ingredients include:

Rhizoma Atractylodis Macrocephalae (*Bai Zhu*)
Radix Albus Paeoniae Lactiflorae (*Bai Shao*)
Pericarpium Citri Reticulatae (*Chen Pi*)
Radix Ledebouriellae Divaricatae (*Fang Feng*)

Within this formula, Atractylodes Macrocephala supplements the spleen and transforms dampness. Peony nourishes the blood and soothes the liver, nourishes the sinews and stops cramping. Pericarpium Citri Reticulatae or Aged Orange Peel rectifies the qi and transforms dampness, while Ledebouriella moves and rectifies the qi both in the small intestine-bladder channels and in the large intestine bowel. It is interesting that so many FMS sufferers also have IBS and that the majority of the FMS diagnostic tender points are on the small intestine and bladder channels. While this formula alone is not sufficient for treating FMS, it is a useful one to take along with other Chinese ready-made medicines.

Xiao Yao Wan

Xiao Yao Wan is used for premenstrual breast distention and pain, premenstrual and menstrual abdominal pain, and chronic constipation from liver depression qi stagnation, particularly in women. It is probably the most commonly prescribed Chinese herbal formula in the world for PMS. It is also used to treat qi stagnation painful menstruation and perimenstrual headache due to a combination of liver depression and blood vacuity. Its Chinese name has been translated as "Free & Easy Pills," "Rambling Pills," "Relaxed Wanderer Pills," and several other versions of this same idea of promoting a freer and smoother, more relaxed flow. As a patent medicine, this formula comes as both pills and desiccated powdered extract. It also dates from the time of William the Conqueror and its ingredients are:

Radix Bupleuri (*Chai Hu*)
Radix Angelicae Sinensis (*Dang Gui*)
Radix Albus Paeoniae Lactiflorae (*Bai Shao*)
Rhizoma Atractylodis Macrocephalae (*Bai Zhu*)
Sclerotium Poriae Cocos (*Fu Ling*)
mix-fried Radix Glycyrrhizae (*Gan Cao*)
Herba Menthae Haplocalycis (*Bo He*)
uncooked Rhizoma Zingiberis (*Sheng Jiang*)

This formula treats the pattern of liver depression qi stagnation complicated by blood vacuity and spleen vacuity with possible dampness as well. Bupleurum courses the liver and rectifies the qi. It is aided in this by Herba Menthae Haplocalycis or Peppermint. Dang Gui and Peony nourish the blood and soften and harmonize the liver. Atractylodes Macrocephala and Poria fortify the spleen and eliminate dampness. Mix-fried Licorice aids these two in fortifying the spleen and supplementing the liver, while Rhizoma Zingiberis or uncooked Ginger aids in both promoting and regulating the qi flow and eliminating dampness.

Because the Bupleurum in the formula can be very drying, it needs to be combined with other ready-made Chinese medicines when cases are complicated by liver blood-kidney yin vacuity as are most cases of FMS. However, when it is combined with other formulas, it can be very useful in helping to manage the liver depression qi stagnation part of FMS.

Dan Zhi Xiao Yao Wan

Dan Zhi Xiao Yao Wan or "Moutan & Gardenia Rambling Pills" is a modification of the above formula which also comes as a patent medicine in the form of pills as well as a desiccated powdered extract. It is meant to treat the pattern of liver depression transforming into heat with spleen vacuity and possible blood vacuity and/or dampness. The ingredients in this formula are the same as above except that two other herbs are added:

Cortex Radicis Moutan (*Dan Pi*)
Fructus Gardeniae Jasminoidis (*Shan Zhi Zi*)

These two ingredients clear heat and resolve depression. In addition, Moutan quickens the blood and dispels stasis and is good at clearing heat specifically from the blood.

Basically, the signs and symptoms of the pattern for which this formula is designed are the same as those for *Xiao Yao Wan* above plus signs and symptoms of depressive heat. These might include a reddish tongue with slightly yellow fur, a bowstring and rapid pulse, a bitter taste in the mouth, and increased irritability. Like Rambling Pills above, this formula can be added to other Chinese ready-made formulas when liver depression and depressive heat are causing significant premenstrual and menstrual complaints.

Suan Zao Ren Tang Wan

This is a pill version of the formula, *Suan Zao Ren Tang* (Zizyphus Seed Decoction). It is also available as a desiccated extract. *Suan Zao Ren Tang* is one of the oldest herbal formulas in Chinese medicine, dating from the second century CE. It treats insomnia and mental unrest due to liver blood vacuity. It can, therefore, be combined with other Chinese ready-made medicines when liver blood vacuity is more severe and manifests primarily as insomnia. Its ingredients are:

Semen Zizyphi Spinosae (*Suan Zao Ren*)
Sclerotium Poriae Cocos (*Fu Ling*)
Radix Ligustici Wallichii (*Chuan Xiong*)
Rhizoma Anemarrhenae Aspheloidis (*Zhi Mu*)
mix-fried Radix Glycyrrhizae (*Gan Cao*)

Within this formula, Zizyphus Spinosa nourishes the heart and liver and quiets the spirit. Poria supplements the spleen and heart, seeps dampness and quiets the heart. Ligusticum Wallichium quickens and move the blood, but especially moves it upward so that it can then nourish the heart and head. In addition, since blood vacuity and blood stasis so commonly go together and, in fact, cause each other, this ingredient promotes the engenderment of new blood through the dispelling of dead or static blood. Anemarrhena clears vacuity heat which may be counterflowing upward to disturb the heart spirit at the same time as it enriches kidney yin. And mix-fried Licorice not only harmonizes all of the other ingredients in this formula but also supplements and nourishes the spleen and heart and, therefore, quiets the heart spirit.

Gui Pi Wan

Gui means to "return or restore," *pi* means "the spleen," and *wan* means "pills." Therefore, the name of these pills means "Restore the Spleen Pills." However, these pills not only supplement the spleen qi but also nourish heart blood and calm the heart spirit. They are the textbook guiding formula for the pattern of heart-spleen dual vacuity. In this case, there are symptoms of spleen qi vacuity, such as fatigue, poor appetite, and cold hands and feet plus symptoms of heart blood vacuity, such as a pale tongue, heart palpitations, impaired memory, confused thinking, and insomnia. This formula is also the standard one for treating heavy or abnormal bleeding due to the spleen not containing and restraining the blood within its vessels. Therefore, this patent medicine can be combined with other Chinese ready-made medicine whenever heart blood and spleen qi vacuity are pronounced. The formula was created by Yan Yong-he in the early 1200s and its ingredients are:

Radix Astragali Membranacei (*Huang Qi*)
Radix Codonopsitis Pilosulae (*Dang Shen*)
Rhizoma Atractylodis Macrocephalae (*Bai Zhu*)
Sclerotium Pararadicis Poriae Cocos (*Fu Shen*)
mix-fried Radix Glycyrrhizae (*Gan Cao*)
Radix Angelicae Sinensis (*Dang Gui*)
Semen Zizyphi Spinosae (*Suan Zao Ren*)
Arillus Euphoriae Longanae (*Long Yan Rou*)
Radix Polygalae Tenuifoliae (*Yuan Zhi*)
Radix Auklandiae Lappae (*Mu Xiang*)

Within this formula, Astragalus, Codonopsis, Atractylodes Macrocephala, Poria, and mix-fried Licorice all supplement the spleen and boost the qi. Poria and Licorice also quiet or calm the spirit. Dang Gui nourishes and quickens the blood. Arillus Longana or Longans also nourishes the blood but specifically heart blood, while Zizyphus Spinosa specifically nourishes liver blood. Polygala rectifies and regulates the qi of the chest. Auklandia rectifies and harmonizes the liver and spleen as well as the stomach and intestinal qi. In addition, it keeps some of the "slimy, enriching" ingredients, such as Dang Gui and Zizyphus Spinosa from damaging the spleen and gumming up the qi mechanism.

Tian Wang Bu Xin Dan

The name of this formula translates as "Heavenly Emperor's Supplement the Heart Elixir." It was created by Hong Ji sometime before 1638. Today, this formula comes as a Chinese patent medicine in pill form and as a desiccated extract. It treats insomnia, restlessness, fatigue, and heart palpitations due to yin, blood, and qi vacuity, with an emphasis on heart yin and liver blood vacuity. It is probably the single most commonly prescribed Chinese formula for insomnia in the Chinese medical repertoire. Its ingredients include:

uncooked Radix Rehmanniae (*Sheng Di*)
Radix Scrophulariae Ningpoensis (*Xuan Shen*)
Fructus Schisandrae Chinensis (*Wu Wei Zi*)
Tuber Asparagi Cochinensis (*Tian Men Dong*)
Tuber Ophiopogonis Japonici (*Mai Men Dong*)
Radix Angelicae Sinensis (*Dang Gui*)
Semen Biotae Orientalis (*Bai Zi Ren*)
Semen Zizyphi Spinosae (*Suan Zao Ren*)
Radix Salviae Miltiorrhizae (*Dan Shen*)
Radix Polygalae Tenuifoliae (*Yuan Zhi*)
Sclerotium Poriae Cocos (*Fu Ling*)
Radix Codonopsitis Pilosulae (*Dang Shen*)

Most of the ingredients in this formula have been described already above. Ophiopogon, Asparagus, Schisandra, and Scrophularia all enrich yin and engender fluids, thus moistening dryness. Scrophularia also clears vacuity heat and scatters phlegm nodulation, Ophiopogon also transforms phlegm and clears heart heat, and Schisandra also has some ability to supplement the chest qi, meaning the heart and lung qi. Biota enriches yin and nourishes the blood as well as moistens the intestines and frees the flow of the stools. This formula can also be combined with other ready-made Chinese medicines when insomnia is a big part of the patient's picture.

An Shen Bu Xin Wan

An shen means "to quiet the spirit." *Bu xin* means "to supplement the heart." Therefore, the Chinese name for these pills means "Quiet the Spirit & Supplement the Heart Pills." This is yet another Chinese patent pill designed to treat insomnia, dizziness, restlessness, profuse dreaming which disturbs the sleep, and heart palpitations due to yin and blood vacuity. Its ingredients also take into account an element of liver depression qi stagnation and an element of phlegm obstruction. In addition, because the ingredient with the largest dose in this formula is Mother of Pearl Powder, this formula helps to downbear upwardly counterflowing yang qi and quiet the spirit quite strongly. Its ingredients are:

Concha Margaritiferae (*Zhen Zhu Mu*)
Radix Polygoni Multiflori (*He Shou Wu*)
Fructus Ligustri Lucidi (*Nu Zhen Zi*)
Herba Ecliptae Prostratae (*Han Lian Cao*)
Semen Cuscutae Chinensis (*Tu Si Zi*)
Fructus Schisandrae Chinensis (*Wu Wei Zi*)
Radix Salviae Miltiorrhizae (*Dan Shen*)
Cortex Albizziae Julibrissin (*He Huan Pi*)
Rhizoma Acori Graminei (*Shi Chang Pu*)

Besides Mother of Pearl, the ingredients in this formula we have not discussed are Polygonum Multiflorum, Ligustrum Lucidum, Eclipta, Cuscuta, Albizzia, and Acorus. Polygonum Multiflorum nourishes the blood in the liver and especially nourishes the sinews. Therefore, it is especially good for muscular stiffness and tingling and numbness of the extremities due to blood vacuity. Ligustrum Lucidum and Eclipta are usually used together. They supplement the liver and kidneys and enrich yin without being "slimy and stagnating." That means they supplement the liver and kidneys without damaging the spleen and creating pathological dampness, a definite consideration in fibromyalgia. Albizzia nourishes the heart and quiets the spirit. It also moves the qi and quickens the blood. Cuscuta supplements the kidneys and invigorates yang. However, it tends to supplement kidney yin and yang evenly. Therefore, it does not typically cause or aggravate vacuity heat. And Acorus transforms phlegm and opens the orifices of the heart when phlegm and dampness are misting or confounding the heart spirit. In many patients with fibromyalgia, the "brain fog" is both due to heart-spleen vacuity and phlegm obstructing the heart spirit.

Once again, this formula may be combined with other appropriate formulas when insomnia plays a large part in fibromyalgia. Because insomnia is such a big part of both the cause and suffering of fibromyalgia syndrome, I have given a number of Chinese herbal medicines that can be used for this extremely uncomfortable and distressing symptom. Insomnia should be one of the very first aspects of this disease the patient and their practitioner should try to bring under control.

Xiang Sha Liu Jun Zi Wan

The name of these pills translates as "Auklandia & Amomum Six Gentlemen Pills." It was created by Zhang Lu-xuan some time before 1695. This formula is currently available in the West as both ready-made pills and powdered extract. It treats the pattern of pronounced spleen vacuity with elements of dampness and qi stagnation effecting primarily the stomach and intestines. These pills are especially good for treating poor appetite, nausea, abdominal bloating after meals, and loose stools due to spleen vacuity and dampness. Their ingredients include:

Radix Codonopsitis Pilosulae (*Dang Shen*)
Rhizoma Atractylodis Macrocephalae (*Bai Zhu*)
Sclerotium Poriae Cocos (*Fu Ling*)
Rhizoma Pinelliae Ternatae (*Ban Xia*)
mix-fried Radix Glycyrrhizae (*Gan Cao*)
Pericarpium Citri Reticulatae (*Chen Pi*)
Radix Auklandiae Lappae (*Mu Xiang*)
Fructus Amomi (*Sha Ren*)

Within this formula, Codonopsis, Atractylodes Macrocephala, Poria, and mix-fried Licorice fortify the spleen and boost the qi. Pinellia and Aged Orange Peel harmonize the stomach and transform phlegm and dampness. Auklandia rectifies and harmonizes the qi of the liver and spleen, stomach and intestines, while Amomum harmonizes the stomach and dries dampness.

One should not take these pills, however, if there are signs of damp heat such as burning around the anus with bowel movements or diarrhea with dark colored, foul-smelling, explosive stools. They can be combined with other Chinese ready-made medicines whenever spleen qi vacuity with dampness and qi stagnation of the stomach and intestines is pronounced.

Bu Zhong Yi Qi Wan

Bu Zhong Yi Qi Wan means "Supplement the Center & Boost the Qi Pills." It is Li Dong-yuan's most famous formula and dates from the time of Genghis Khan. This formula is available from a wide variety of suppliers in both pill and powdered extract form. It treats the pattern of central qi vacuity or central qi downward fall. The central qi is another name for the spleen and stomach qi. This formula is especially good for treating spleen vacuity weakness manifesting not so much as digestive complaints and diarrhea but as more pronounced fatigue and orthostatic hypotension. Orthostatic hypotension means dizziness on standing up. The ingredients in this formula are:

Radix Astragali Membranacei (*Huang Qi*)
Radix Codonopsitis Pilosulae (*Dang Shen*)
Rhizoma Atractylodis Macrocephalae (*Bai Zhu*)
mix-fried Radix Glycyrrhizae (*Gan Cao*)
Radix Angelicae Sinensis (*Dang Gui*)
Radix Bupleuri (*Chai Hu*)
Rhizoma Cimicifugae (*Sheng Ma*)
Pericarpium Citri Reticulatae (*Chen Pi*)
Fructus Zizyphi Jujubae (*Da Zao*)
uncooked Rhizoma Zingiberis (*Sheng Jiang*)

This is actually a very sophisticated formula and it has a very wide range of application. It can be added to other formulas when spleen vacuity causing fatigue is more pronounced. Within this formula, Astragalus, Codonopsis, Atractylodes Macrocephala, and mix-fried Licorice strongly fortify the spleen and boost the qi. Dang Gui nourishes the blood. Since blood is the mother of the qi, the addition of this ingredient in this formula actually helps supplement the qi more effectively. Bupleurum and Cimicifuga course the liver and rectify the qi, upbear the clear and, therefore, promote downbearing of the turbid as well as fortification of the spleen. Aged Orange Peel and uncooked Ginger both harmonize the stomach, downbear turbidity, and transform phlegm and dampness. Zizyphus Jujuba or Red Dates supplement the spleen and nourish the heart. In addition, mix-fried Licorice and Red Dates quiet the heart spirit.

Yu Ping Feng San Wan

This formula was created by Zhu Dan-xi also around the time of Genghis Khan. Its name means "Jade Windscreen Powder Pills." It is meant for a defensive qi vacuity with easy invasion by external evils. Its ingredients are:

Radix Astragali Membranacei (*Huang Qi*)
Rhizoma Atractylodes Macrocephalae (*Bai Zhu*)
Radix Ledebouriellae Divaricatae (*Fang Feng*)

The ruling medicinal in this formula is Astragalus which strongly supplements the spleen and, therefore, also the lung and defensive qi. It is aided by Atractylodes Macrocephala which also supplements the spleen. However, Atractylodes also transforms dampness, and dampness often plays a role in fibromyalgia. Ledebouriella is an exterior-resolving medicinal which gently removes any lingering pathogens in the exterior layers of the body. However, it also treats wind damp impediment pain in the small intestine and bladder channels where most of the tender points of fibromyalgia are located. This formula comes as both pills and powdered extracts. It can be combined with other Chinese ready-made medicines whenever there is a tendency to recurrent infections and allergies. However, it is for the prevention of infections and allergies and does not treat allergies and infections per se. During an allergic attack or during an infection, other Chinese medicines should be used. For more information on the Chinese medical treatment of hayfever and asthma, please see my *Curing Hayfever Naturally with Chinese Medicine* also available from Blue Poppy Press.

Yi Guan Jian Wan

The name of this formula translates as "One Link Decoction Pills." It was created by Wei Zhi-xiu at around the time of the American revolution in the eighteenth century. It is meant for the treatment of liver blood-kidney yin vacuity with liver depression qi stagnation. Its ingredients include:

uncooked Radix Rehmanniae (*Sheng Di*)
Fructus Lycii Chinensis (*Gou Qi Zi*)
Radix Angelicae Sinensis (*Dang Gui*)
Radix Glehniae Littoralis (*Sha Shen*)
Tuber Ophiopogonis Japonicae (*Mai Dong*)
Fructus Meliae Toosendan (*Chuan Lian Zi*)

Within this formula, uncooked Rehmannia nourishes, cools, and quickens the blood. Dang Gui also nourishes and quickens the blood. Rehmannia supplements the yin of the kidneys, while Dang Gui supplements the blood of the liver. Fructus Lycii Chinensis also supplements kidney yin at the same time as it nourishes liver blood. Glehnia and Ophiopogon both enrich yin and engender fluids. And Melia courses the liver and rectifies the qi. Since Melia also kills parasites and "parasites" in Chinese medicine are typically associated with damp heat, Melia is a good qi-rectifying medicinal to use when there is the complication of damp heat. Also, because it does not damage and consume yin fluids the way Bupleurum does, it is a good qi-rectifying medicinal to use when there is yin vacuity.

This formula now comes in both pill and powdered extract forms. It can be combined with other Chinese ready-made medicines whenever liver blood-kidney yin vacuity and liver depression qi stagnation are more pronounced.

Da Bu Yin Wan

This is another of Zhu Dan-xi's famous formulas created sometime in the thirteenth century. Its name means "Greatly

Supplementing Yin Pills." It is available both as pills and powdered extract. It is designed to treat yin vacuity with vacuity heat. Its ingredients are:

cooked Radix Rehmanniae (*Shu Di*)
Plastrum Testudinis (*Gui Ban*)
Cortex Phellodendri (*Huang Bai*)
Rhizoma Anemarrhenae Aspheloidis (*Zhi Mu*)

Within this formula, cooked Rehmannia nourishes the blood and supplements yin. It is assisted in these functions by Plastrum Testudinis which also strongly enriches yin. However, Plastrum Testudinis (the under shell of a species of turtle) represses upward counterflowing yang, quickens and frees the flow of the network vessels, and also has some ability to treat damp heat. Phellodendron and Anemarrhena are a commonly combined pair of Chinese medicinals for vacuity heat. Phellodendron clears vacuity heat in the upper body and damp heat in the lower body. Anemarrhena clears heat and enriches kidney yin. Therefore, this medicine can be combined with other Chinese ready-made medicines whenever yin vacuity with vacuity heat is more pronounced. Because cooked Rehmannia can either cause or worsen diarrhea, this medicine should not be taken if there are loose stools or diarrhea.

Shou Wu Pian

Shou Wu Pian means "Polygonum Multiflorum Tablets" and these tablets are made out of this single Chinese herbal ingredient, Radix Polygoni Multiflori (*He Shou Wu*). This medicinal strongly nourishes liver blood and enriches kidney yin, with an emphasis on liver blood. Therefore, it is an excellent medicinal for treating malnourishment of the sinews with muscular stiffness and numbness and tingling of the extremities. Available as a pill or capsule, this medicine can be combined with other Chinese ready-made medicines whenever liver blood vacuity is more pronounced. This medicinal also has some spirit-quieting or sedative abilities and may even help regulate the flora and fauna in the intestinal tract. One whole school of Chinese medicine considers this an important supplementing herb whenever there are complex, multi-pattern conditions associated with intestinal tract problems.

Huan Shao Dan Wan

The name of this medicine translates as "Restore Lesser (Years) Elixir Pills." It is an ancient Chinese folk formula which now comes as both pills and powdered extract. It treats a combination of kidney yin and yang vacuity complicated by some spleen qi vacuity. In pill form, its ingredients are:

cooked Radix Rehmanniae (*Shu Di*)
Fructus Lycii Chinensis (*Gou Qi Zi*)
Rhizoma Dioscoreae Hypoglaucae (*Bi Xie*)
Sclerotium Poriae Cocos (*Fu Ling*)
Herba Cistanchis Deserticolae (*Rou Cong Rong*)
Fructus Foeniculi Vulgaris (*Xiao Hui Xiang*)
Radix Morindae Officinalis (*Ba Ji Tian*)
Cortex Eucommiae Ulmoidis (*Du Zhong*)
Radix Achyranthis Bidentatae (*Niu Xi*)
Fructus Schisandrae Chinensis (*Wu Wei Zi*)
Fructus Zizyphi Jujubae (*Da Zao*)
Fructus Corni Officinalis (*Shan Zhu Yu*)
Fructus Broussonetiae (*Zhu Shi Zi*)

Cooked Rehmannia, Lycium, Achyranthes, and Broussonetia supplement liver blood and kidney yin. Broussonetia also clears liver channel heat, while Achyranthes has some ability to quicken the blood and lead upwardly counterflowing yang back downward to its source in the lower half of the body. Cistanches, Morinda, and Eucommia all nourish liver blood at the same time as they invigorate or strengthen kidney yang. Achyranthes, Eucommia, and Morinda all also specifically strengthen the sinews and the bones. Poria supplements the spleen qi at the same time as it seeps dampness, while Dioscorea Hypoglauca seeps dampness and treats wind damp impediment pain. Cornus supplements both kidney yin and kidney yang in a balanced or even way. Schisandra, like Cornus, is categorized as an astringent herb, but both medicinals also have an ability to supplement the kidney qi. Foeniculum or Fennel moves the qi in the liver channel, and Red Dates harmonize the rest of the medicinals in this formula as well as supplement spleen qi and heart blood.

When kidney yang complicates fibromyalgia, there is also usually spleen qi vacuity, blood and/or yin vacuity, and some sort of heat. Therefore, this formula can be combined with other ready-made Chinese medicines when kidney yang complicates these other patterns. Because it is well-balanced within itself and does not use medicinals that are excessively warm, it will not aggravate either damp, depressive, or vacuity heat when combined with other medicines which include ingredients for clearing heat.

Where to order the above medicines

The pill forms of the above Chinese patent medicines can be ordered directly from either of two companies:

Mayway Corp.
1338 Mandela Parkway
Oakland, CA 94607 USA
Tel: 1-800-2-MAYWAY
Fax: 1-800-909-2828
e-mail: sales@mayway.com
Website: www.mayway.com

Nuherbs Co.
3820 Penniman Ave.
Oakland, CA 94619 USA
Tel: 510-534-4372
    800-233-4307
Fax: 510-534-4384
    800-550-1928

Desiccated powdered extracts of the above Chinese medicinal formulas are available from:

Qualiherb/Finemost Corp.
13340 E. Firestone Blvd. #N
Santa Fe Springs, CA 90670 USA
Tel: 1-800-533-5907

Side effects

The above Chinese patent medicines only give a suggestion of how one or several over-the-counter Chinese ready-made medicines may be used to treat FMS. As a professional practitioner of Chinese medicine, I prefer to see people receive a professional diagnosis and an individually tailored prescription. However, as long as one is careful to try to match up their pattern with the right formula and not to exceed the recommended dosage on each medicine's package, one can try treating their FMS with one or more of these remedies. If it works, great! These patent medicines are usually quite cheap compared to Western prescription drugs. If this approach doesn't work after three months or if there are *any side effects*, one should stop and see a professional practitioner.

In general, you can tell if any medication and treatment are good for you by checking the following six guideposts.

1. Digestion
2. Elimination
3. Energy level

4. Mood
5. Appetite
6. Sleep

If a medication, be it modern Western or traditional Chinese, gets rid of your symptoms and all six of these basic areas of human health improve or are fine to begin with, then that medicine or treatment is probably OK. However, even if a treatment or medication takes away your major complaint, if it causes deterioration in one of these six basic parameters, then that treatment or medication is probably not OK and is certainly not OK for long–term use. When medicines and treatments, even so-called natural, herbal medications, are prescribed based on a person's pattern of disharmony, then there is healing without side effects. According to Chinese medicine, this is the only kind of true healing.

10
Acupuncture & Moxibustion

When the average Westerner thinks of Chinese medicine, they probably first think of acupuncture. Certainly acupuncture is the best known of the various methods of treatment which go to make up Chinese medicine. However, in China, acupuncture is actually a secondary treatment modality, most Chinese immediately thinking of "herbal"[1] medicine when thinking of Chinese medicine.

Be that as it may, most professional practitioners of Chinese medicine in North America are licensed or otherwise registered and permitted to practice medicine as acupuncturists. Therefore, most practitioners treat every patient with at least some acupuncture no matter if they also prescribe a Chinese herbal formula as well. While this "doubling up" of these two therapies is not always necessary to successfully treat FMS, FMS in general does respond very well to correctly prescribed and administered acupuncture.

What is acupuncture?

Acupuncture primarily means the insertion of extremely thin, sterilized, stainless steel needles into specific points on the body where Chinese doctors have known for centuries there are special concentrations of qi and blood. Therefore, these points are like switches or circuit breakers for regulating and balancing the flow of qi and blood over the channel and network system we described above. As we have seen, because FMS always involves

---

[1] The ingredients in Chinese medicines can be animal, vegetable, or mineral and thus it is not precisely accurate to call them "herbal".

pain, it also always involves a lack of free flow of the qi and/or blood. Because it is a chronic, frustrating problem, it also always involves liver depression qi stagnation. Since acupuncture's forte is the regulation and rectification of the flow of qi (and, thus secondarily, the blood), it is an especially good treatment mode for correcting diseases characterized by pain and/or associated with liver depression qi stagnation. In that case, insertion of acupuncture needles at various points in the body moves stagnant qi in the liver and leads the qi to flow in its proper directions and amounts.

As a generic term, acupuncture also includes several other methods of stimulating acupuncture points, thus regulating the flow of qi in the body. The main other modality is moxibustion. This means the warming of acupuncture points mainly by burning dried, aged Oriental mugwort on, near, or over acupuncture points. The purpose of this warming treatment are to 1) even more strongly stimulate the flow of qi and blood, 2) add warmth to areas of the body which are too cold, and 3) add yang qi to the body to supplement a yang qi deficiency. Other acupuncture modalities are to apply suction cups over points, to massage the points, to prick the points to allow a drop or two of blood to exit, to apply Chinese medicinals to the points, to apply magnets to the points, and to stimulate the points by either electricity or laser.

What is a typical acupuncture treatment for FMS like?

In China, acupuncture treatments are given every day or every other day. After a course of 10 treatments there is a break of a few days and then another course of 10 treatments is started. In the United States, some practitioners will treat two or three times in a week in the beginning of a case or if there are really acute symptoms, but most treat once a week. When acupuncture is combined with Chinese herbal medicine, this more relaxed treatment schedule seems to work OK.

When a person comes for an appointment, the practitioner will ask what the main symptoms are, will typically look at the tongue and its fur, and will feel the pulses at the radial arteries on both wrists. Then, they will ask the patient to lie down on a treatment table. Based on their Chinese pattern discrimination, the practitioner will select anywhere from a couple to a dozen points to be needled.

The needles used today are ethylene oxide gas sterilized disposable needles. This means that they are used one time and then thrown away, just like a hypodermic syringe in a doctor's office. However, unlike relatively fat hypodermic needles, acupuncture needles are hardly thicker than a strand of hair. The skin over the point is disinfected with alcohol and the needle is quickly and deftly inserted somewhere typically between one sixteenth to one half an inch. In some few cases, a needle may be inserted deeper than that, but most needles are only inserted relatively shallowly.

After the needle has broken the skin, the acupuncturist will usually manipulate the needle in various ways until he or she feels that the qi has "arrived." This refers to a subtle but very real feeling of resistance around the needle. When the qi arrives, the patient will usually feel a mild, dull soreness around the needle, a slight electrical feeling, a heavy feeling, or a numb or tingly feeling. All these mean that the needle has tapped the qi and that treatment will be effective. Once the qi has been tapped, then the practitioner may further adjust the qi flow by manipulating the needle in certain ways, may attach the needle to an electro-acupuncture machine in order to stimulate the point with very mild and gentle electricity, or they may simply leave the needle in place. Usually the needles are left in place from 10-20 minutes. After this, the needles are withdrawn and thrown away. *Thus there is absolutely no chance for cross-infection from another patient.*

How are the points selected?

The points one's acupuncturist chooses to needle each treatment are selected on the basis of Chinese medical theory and the known clinical effects of certain points. Since there are different schools or styles of acupuncture, point selection tends to vary from practitioner to practitioner. However, let me present a fairly typical case from the point of view of the dominant style of acupuncture in the People's Republic of China.

Let's take Hannah again as our example. Hannah's pattern was a qi and yin vacuity with damp heat impediment, liver depression, and blood. Her main symptoms were muscle-joint aching and pain, insomnia, fatigue, and PMS. The treatment principles necessary for remedying this case are to fortify the spleen and boost the qi, nourish the liver and enrich the kidneys, free the flow of impediment and stop pain, course the liver and rectify the qi, and quicken the blood and dispel stasis.[2] Because insomnia is such an important symptom in Hannah's case, I am also going to add the principle of quieting the spirit which will then promote better sleep. In order to accomplish these aims, the practitioner might select the following points:

Zu San Li (Stomach 36)	*Qu Quan* (Liver 8)
San Yin Jiao (Spleen 6)	*Nei Guan* (Pericardium 6)
Xue Hai (Spleen 10)	*Shen Men* (Heart 7)
Tai Xi (Kidney 3)	*Hou Xi* (Small Intestine 3)
Tai Chong (Liver 3)	*Shen Mai* (Bladder 62)

In this case, Stomach 36 and Spleen 6 are meant to fortify the spleen and boost the qi. However, Stomach 36 will also treat any pain located anywhere along the course of the stomach channel and even somewhat along the course of the large intestine

---

[2] The reader may ask why there are no treatment principles for the damp heat pattern in this list. This is because I am going to treat the damp heat component of Hannah's diagnosis primarily by herbs and diet. There are no special acupuncture needling techniques for damp heat impediment as opposed to any other type of impediment.

channel, since these two are connected. Spleen 6 also supplements and regulates the liver and kidneys, since all three channels cross at this point, and it also regulates menstruation and urination since all three of those channels enter the lower abdomen. Kidney 3 supplements the kidneys and enriches yin. This effect is even stronger when Kidney 3 is combined with Spleen 6. Liver 8 nourishes liver blood. Liver 3 courses the liver and rectifies the qi. Spleen 10 is a special point associated with the blood. Although some people say it supplements the blood, I believe it primarily quickens the blood and dispels stasis. Interestingly, it is one of the 18 diagnostic tender points for fibromyalgia! Pericardium 6 and Heart 7 are a commonly used pair for quieting the spirit and promoting deep and continuous sleep.

The last two points are my own special method for treating fibromylagia. These two points are located on the small intestine and bladder channels which together form a single pathway called the *tai yang* or greatest yang. The *tai yang* channels run up the back side of the arms and legs and up the back, over the neck and shoulders, and down onto the cheeks. A majority of the 18 tender points of fibromyalgia are located on this *tai yang* pathway. These two points are ruling or main points for dealing with pain along the course of these two channels. However, these two points are also a pair of points which control another channel called the *du mai* or governing vessel. This channel runs up the back directly over the center of the spine.

In the thirteenth century, around the time of Genghis and Kublai Khan, Li Dong-yuan and Zhu Dan-xi were considered two of the greatest Chinese doctors of their day. These two doctors developed a theory within Chinese medicine called yin fire theory. This theory is an explanation of complex, multi-pattern conditions causing "knotty, difficult to treat diseases" where there is a combination of spleen vacuity, liver depression, and some kind of heat, whether damp, depressive, and/or vacuity. According to this theory, if there is spleen vacuity, liver depression, and one or more of the three above kinds of heat, this heat will float upward to accumulate in the heart. On the one hand, this heat disturbs the heart spirit giving rise to symptoms of anxiety, agitation, restlessness, irritability, insomnia, and heart palpitations. However, this heat is often also passed from the heart to its yang paired channel, the small intestine, and also to the governing vessel. Once inside the small intestine, this counterflowing heat may then flow into the bladder channel and even into the gallbladder channel located right next to it. When such counterflowing yang qi flows into these channels where it is not supposed to be, it causes blockage and impediment to the qi and blood flowing in these channels. This theory explains the overwhelming majority of the 18 fibromyalgia tender points which are located on the small intestine, bladder, and gallbladder channels.[3] It is also why I always use Small Intestine 3 and Bladder 62 in my acupuncture treatment of fibromyalgia patients.

Depending on the patient's other signs and symptoms at the time of treatment, other points might also be chosen. For instance, if there was diarrhea, *Tian Shu* (Stomach 25) and *Da Chang Shu* (Bladder 25), two points with a direct connection to the large intestine, might be added. If there was headache, points on the head might be added. If there was severe insomnia, *Bai Hui* (Governing Vessel 20) and *An Mian Xue* (a special non-channel point for insomnia) might be added to more strongly improve the sleep.

So far, the acupuncture I have described is mostly designed to treat the underlying disease mechanisms but has not addressed the muscle-joint aching and pain per se. For this, I personally recommend needling all points painful to pressure with a very shallow insertion using what is technically called sparrow-pecking technique. This is a very slight up and down motion with the needle after it has pierced the skin. This is done just after the needle has gone through the skin and fat but before it enters the body of the underlying muscles. Although this technique may sound painful, in actual fact, the patient usually feels nothing at

---

[3] The few others are located on the stomach and large intestine channels.

all after the quick insertion through the skin. This same man-euver is done at as many of the 18 tender points as are actually painful that day, using a single needle and moving from tender point to tender point without leaving these needles in place. In other words, this technique is done on all tender points while the needles in the other main or ruling points are being passively left in place. The good news is that there should be less and less tender points with each successive treatment.

When using the above combination of ruling and auxiliary tender points for fibromyalgia, I typically recommend one treatment per week for four weeks, then another two treatments spaced two weeks apart, and a single last treatment at the end of the third month. Thus, for fibromylagia, I commonly do a total of seven treatments over three months. At the end of this time, not only has the bodily aching and pain improved, but sleep is better, mood is better, digestion and elimination are better, urination is not so urgent and frequent, TMJ and bruxism have disappeared, and even allergies and sinusitis have disappeared. After these initial seven treatments, I then tell my patients to come back in for "brush-ups" after six months as necessary. When such acupuncture is combined with Chinese herbal medicine and proper diet, relaxation, and exercise, it is extremely effective.

Does acupuncture hurt?

In Chinese, it is said that acupuncture is *bu tong*, painless. However, most patients will feel some mild soreness, heaviness, electrical tingling, or distention. When done well and sensitively, it should not be sharp, biting, burning, or really painful and most people experience very little discomfort at all.

How quickly will I feel the result?

One of the best things about the acupuncture treatment of FMS is that its effects are immediate. Since many of the symptoms of FMS have to do with stuck qi, as soon as the qi is made to flow, the symptoms disappear. Therefore, when treating a number of

FMS complaints, such as body pain, abdominal cramps, and headache, *one will feel relief during the treatment itself.*

In addition, because feelings of being "stressed out" and nervous tension are also mostly due to liver depression qi stagnation, most people will feel an immediate relief of stress and tension while still on the table. Typically, one will feel a pronounced tranquility and relaxation within five to ten minutes of the insertion of the needles.

Who should get acupuncture?

As mentioned above, because most professional practitioners in the West are legally entitled to practice under various acupuncture laws, most acupuncturists will routinely do acupuncture on every patient. Since acupuncture's effects on FMS are usually so immediate, this is usually a good thing for FMS sufferers. Because acupuncture treats pain so effectively and immediately, one should definitely consider receiving acupunc-ture for any FMS complaints associated with pain. And because acupuncture treats mental-emotional tension so well and so immediately, those with these types of symptoms should also get at least one course of acupuncture therapy.

However, when FMS symptoms mostly have to do with qi, blood, and yin vacuities, then acupuncture is not as effective as internally administered Chinese herbal medicinals. Although moxibustion can add yang qi to the body (and I will teach a home remedy for this in a separate section on moxibustion below), acupuncture needles cannot add qi, blood, or yin to a body in short supply of these. The best acupuncture can do in these cases is to stimulate the various viscera and bowels which engender and transform the qi, blood, and yin. Chinese herbs, on the other hand, can directly introduce qi, blood, and yin-building substances into the body, thus immediately supplementing these types of vacuities. In FMS cases where qi, blood, and yin vacuities are pronounced, one should either use acupuncture with Chinese medicinals or rely on Chinese medicinals alone.

Ear acupuncture

Acupuncturists believe there is a map of the entire body in the ear and that by stimulating the corresponding points in the ear, one can remedy those areas and functions of the body. Therefore, many acupuncturists will not only needle points on the body at large but also select one or more points on the ear. In terms of FMS, needling the ear point *Shen Men* (Spirit Gate) can have a profound effect on relaxing tension and irritability and improving sleep. There are also ear points for the liver, spleen, stomach, and large intestine and all the muscles and joints of the body.

The nice thing about ear acupuncture points is that one can use tiny "press needles" which are shaped like miniature thumbtacks. These are pressed into the points, covered with adhesive tape, and left in place for five to seven days. This method can provide continuous treatment between regularly scheduled office visits. Hence ear acupuncture is a nice way of extending the duration of an acupuncture treatment. In addition, these ear points can also be stimulated with small metal pellets, radish seeds, or tiny magnets, thus getting the benefits of stimulating these points without having to insert actual needles.

11
The Three Free Therapies

Although one can experiment cautiously with Chinese herbal medicinals, one cannot really do acupuncture on oneself. Therefore, Chinese herbal medicine and acupuncture and its related modalities mostly require the aid of a professional practitioner. However, there are three free therapies which are crucial to preventing and treating FMS. These are diet, exercise, and deep relaxation.

Remember that the root causes of FMS are qi and blood vacuities, damp heat impediment, and qi stagnation and blood stasis. However, also remember that impediment is nothing other than stasis and stagnation. The term impediment simply means a lack of free flow mainly in the extremities. Of these three free therapies, diet is designed to treat the spleen and, therefore, cure the qi and blood vacuities, while exercise and relaxation are meant to cure the qi and blood stasis and stagnation. When all three are coordinated, they thus eliminate the causes and disease mechanisms of FMS. Since Western diets are, by Chinese medical standards, typically poor and since Western society tends to be both excessively sedentary and excessively stressful, lack of proper management of these three basic realms of human life is the reason why so many people in the West suffer from FMS. In other words, although FMS has been around for millennia, its incidence is probably higher now in the West because of relatively recent changes in our diet and lifestyle.

Diet

As discussed earlier, in Chinese medicine, the function of the spleen and stomach are likened to a pot on a stove or still. The stomach receives the foods and liquids which then "rotten and ripen" like a mash in a fermentation vat. The spleen then cooks this mash and drives off (*i.e.,* transforms and upbears) the pure part. This pure part collects in the lungs to become the qi and in the heart to become the blood. In addition, Chinese medicine characterizes this transformation as a process of yang qi transforming yin substance. All the principles of Chinese dietary therapy, including what people with FMS should and should not eat, are derived from these basic "facts."

We have seen that a healthy spleen is vitally important for keeping the liver in check and the qi freely flowing. We have also seen that the spleen is the root of qi and blood transformation and engenderment. If the qi and blood production is healthy and abundant, then the sinews and bones will be nourished and the defensive qi will protect against invasion of the body by any pathogens. In addition, there will be a surplus of qi and blood, and this surplus will be converted into yin essence stored in and used to bolster and support the kidneys. Therefore, it is vitally important for those with FMS to avoid foods which damage the spleen and to eat foods which promote a healthy spleen and qi and blood production.

Foods which damage the spleen

In terms of foods which damage the spleen, Chinese medicine begins with uncooked, chilled foods. If the process of digestion is likened to cooking, then cooking is nothing other than predigestion outside of the body. In Chinese medicine, it is a given that the overwhelming majority of all food should be cooked, *i.e.,* predigested. Although cooking may destroy some vital nutrients (in Chinese, qi), cooking does render the remaining nutrients much more easily assimilable. Therefore, even though some nutrients have been lost, the net absorption of nutrients is greater with cooked foods than raw. Further, eating raw foods makes the spleen work harder and thus wears the spleen out more quickly. If one's spleen is very robust, eating uncooked, raw foods may not be so damaging, but we have already seen that in FMS sufferers, the spleen is almost always already weak.

More importantly, chilled foods directly damage the spleen. Chilled, frozen foods and drinks neutralize the spleen's yang qi. The process of digestion is the process of warming all foods and drinks to 100° Fahrenheit (38° C) within the stomach so that it may undergo transformation. If the spleen expends too much yang qi just warming the food up, then it will become damaged and weak. Therefore, all foods and liquids should be eaten and drunk at room temperature at the least and better at body temperature. The more signs and symptoms of spleen vacuity a person presents, such as fatigue, chronically loose stools, undigested food in the stools, cold hands and feet, dizziness on standing up, and aversion to cold, the more important it is to avoid uncooked, chilled foods and drinks.

In addition, sugars and sweets directly damage the spleen. This is because sweet is the flavor which inherently "enters" the spleen. It is also an inherently dampening flavor according to Chinese medicine. This means that the body engenders or secretes fluids which gather and collect, transforming into dampness, in response to foods with an excessively sweet flavor. In Chinese medicine, it is said that the spleen is averse to dampness. Dampness is yin and controls or checks yang qi. The spleen's function is based on the transformative and transporting functions of yang qi. Therefore, anything which is excessively dampening can damage the spleen. The sweeter a food is, the more dampening and, therefore, more damaging it is to the spleen.

Another group of foods which are dampening and, therefore, damaging to the spleen is what Chinese doctors call "sodden wheat foods." This means flour products such as bread and noodles. Wheat, as opposed to rice, is damp by nature. When wheat is steamed, yeasted, and/or refined, it becomes even more dampening. In addition, all oils and fats are damp by nature and, hence, may damage the spleen. The more oily or greasy a food is, the worse it is for the spleen. Because milk contains a lot of fat, dairy products are another spleen-damaging, dampness-engendering food. This includes milk, butter, and cheese.

If we put this all together, then ice cream is just about the worst thing a person with a weak, damp spleen could eat. Ice cream is chilled, it is intensely sweet, and it is filled with fat. Therefore, it is a triple whammy when it comes to damaging the spleen. Likewise, pasta smothered in tomato sauce and cheese is a recipe for disaster. Pasta made from wheat flour is dampening, tomatoes are dampening, and cheese is dampening. In addition, what many people don't know is that a glass of fruit juice contains as much sugar as a candy bar, and, therefore, is also very damp-engendering and damaging to the spleen.

Below is a list of specific Western foods which damage the spleen because they are either uncooked, chilled, too sweet, or too dampening. In people with FMS, consumption of these foods should be minimized or avoided in proportion to the degree of weakness and dampness of the spleen.

Ice cream
Sugar
Candy, especially chocolate
Milk
Butter
Cheese
Margarine
Yogurt
Raw salads
Fruit juices

Juicy, sweet fruits, such as
   oranges, peaches,
   strawberries, and tomatoes
Fatty meats
Fried foods
Refined flour products
Yeasted bread
Nuts
Alcohol (which is essentially
   sugar)

If the spleen is weak and wet, one should also not eat too much at any one time. A weak spleen can be overwhelmed by a large meal, especially if any of the food is hard-to-digest. This then results in food stagnation which only impedes the free flow of qi all the more and further damages the spleen.

A clear, bland diet

In Chinese medicine, the best diet for the spleen and, therefore, by extension for most humans, is what is called a "clear, bland diet." This is a diet high in complex carbohydrates such as unrefined grains, especially rice, and beans. It is a diet which is high in *lightly cooked* vegetables. It is a diet which is low in fatty meats, oily, greasy, fried foods, and very sweet foods. However, it is not a completely vegetarian diet. Most people, in my experience should eat one to two ounces of various types of meat two to four times per week. This animal flesh may be the highly popular but overtouted chicken and fish, but should also include some lean beef, pork, and lamb. Since most FMS patients exhibit a blood and/or yin vacuity and animal products are considered supplementing to the blood and yin, FMS sufferers usually need some animal foods in their diets. However, since animal foods are hard to digest and most FMS sufferers have weak spleens, one should be careful not to eat too much meat and animal products. Some fresh or cooked fruits may be eaten, but fruit juices should be avoided. In addition, one should make an effort to include tofu and tempeh, two soy foods now commonly available in North American grocery food stores.

If the spleen is weak, then one should eat several smaller meals rather than one or two large meals. In addition, because rice is 1) neutral in temperature, 2) it fortifies the spleen and supplements the qi, and 3) it eliminates dampness, rice should be the main or staple grain in the diet.

101

A few problem foods

There are a few "problem" foods which deserve special mention. The first of these is coffee. Many people crave coffee for two reasons. First, coffee moves stuck qi. Therefore, in a person who suffers from liver depression qi stagnation, coffee will temporarily provide the feeling that the qi is flowing. Secondly, coffee transforms essence into qi and makes that qi temporarily available to the body. Therefore, those who suffer from spleen and/or kidney vacuity fatigue will get a temporary lift from coffee. They will feel like they have energy. However, once this energy is used up, they are left with a negative deficit. The coffee has transformed some of the essence stored in the kidneys into qi. This qi has been used, and now there is less stored essence. Since the blood and essence share a common source, coffee drinking may ultimately worsen any symptoms of FMS associated with blood or kidney vacuities.

Another problem food is chocolate. Chocolate is a combination of oil, sugar, and cocoa. We have seen that both oil and sugar are dampening and damaging to the spleen. Temporarily, the sugar will boost the spleen qi, but ultimately it will result in "sugar blues" or a hypoglycemic let-down. Cocoa stirs the life gate fire. The life gate fire is another name for kidney yang or kidney fire, and kidney fire is the source of sexual energy and desire. It is said that chocolate is the food of love, and from the Chinese medical point of view, that is true. Since chocolate stimulates kidney fire at the same time as it temporarily boosts the spleen, it does give one rush of yang qi. In addition, this rush of yang qi does move depression and stagnation, at least short-term. So it makes sense that some people with liver depression, spleen vacuity, and kidney yang debility might crave chocolate. However, chocolate ultimately damages the spleen and engenders damp heat and this, in turn, may aggravate yin vacuity and vacuity heat.

Alcohol is both damp and hot according to Chinese medical theory. It strongly moves the qi and blood. Therefore, persons with liver depression qi stagnation will feel temporarily better from drinking alcohol. However, the sugar in alcohol damages the spleen and engenders dampness which "gums up the works," while the heat (yang) in alcohol can waste the blood (yin) and aggravate or inflame depressive liver heat.

Spicy, peppery, "hot" foods also move the qi, thereby giving some temporary relief to liver depression qi stagnation. However, like alcohol, the heat in spicy hot foods wastes the blood and can inflame yang.

In Chinese medicine, the sour flavor is inherently astringing and constricting. Therefore, people with FMS should limit their intake of vinegar and other intensely sour foods. Such sour-flavored foods may aggravate the qi stagnation by astringing and restricting the qi and blood all the more. This is also why sweet and sour foods, such as orange juice and tomatoes are particularly bad for those with liver depression/spleen vacuity. The sour flavor astringes and constricts the qi, while the sweet flavor damages the spleen and engenders dampness.

Candidiasis & FMS

Dr. Roger L. Turner, a chiropractor in Toronto, Canada who specializes in treating fibromyalgia, says that many patients with this condition also suffer from candidiasis.[1] If one looks at the foods which I have recommended to minimize or avoid above and what I have recommended to eat, one will see that it comes very close or is identical to an anti-candida diet. Polysystemic chronic candidiasis (PSCC) refers to a chronic overgrowth of yeasts and fungi in the body which then goes on to affect many different systems in the body. The pathological changes associated with PSCC are due to a combination of food allergies, immune system

---

[1] Turner, Roger L, www.vianet.on.ca/comm/wellness/fibromyalgia 1.htm

dysregulation, and autoimmune reactions. These pathological changes may affect the adrenals, pituitary gland, and thyroid gland, and in women, the ovaries. In the West, a tendency towards PSCC is due to faulty diet as outlined above, overuse of antibiotics, and overuse of hormone-based medicine from oral birth control pills to corticosteroids. From a Chinese medical point of view, this then results in deep-seated spleen vacuity with damp encumbrance usually complicated by liver depression and possibly by phlegm fluids, damp heat, and/or blood stasis in addition. Kidney yang vacuity may also develop if the spleen vacuity goes on for long enough or simply as a result of aging.

If a person with FMS has a history of multiple fungal and yeast infections, a history of recurrent or enduring antibiotic use (such as for recurrent bladder infections, acne, or pelvic inflammatory disease), has a history of hormones used as medicine, or suffers from allergies, PSCC should be suspected as a component of that person's FMS. In that case, it is necessary to pay particular attention to the diet. The good news is that professionally prescribed Chinese herbal medicine can help remedy PSCC faster than just diet alone. The bad news is that, without proper diet, no amount of Chinese herbs will completely and permanently remedy this condition.

Some last words on diet

In conclusion, there are no magic foods that cure FMS. Diet most definitely plays a major role in the cause and perpetuation of FMS, but the issue is mainly what to avoid or minimize, not what to eat. Most of us know that coffee, chocolate, sugars and sweets, oils and fats, and alcohol are not good for us. Most of us know that we should be eating more complex carbohydrates and freshly cooked vegetables and less fatty meats. However, it's one thing to know these things and another to follow what we know.

To be perfectly honest, a clear bland diet *à la* Chinese medicine is not the most exciting diet in the world. It is the traditional diet of most lower and lower middle class peoples around the world living in temperate climates. It is the traditional diet of most of my readers' great grandparents. The point I am making here is that our modern Western diet which is high in oils and fats, high in sugars and sweets, high in animal proteins, and proportionally high in uncooked, chilled foods and drinks is a relatively recent aberration, and you can't fool Mother Nature.

When one switches to the clear, bland diet of Chinese medicine, at first one may suffer from cravings for more "flavorful" food. These cravings are, in many cases, actually associated with food "allergies." In other words, we may crave what is actually not good for us similar to an alcoholic craving alcohol. After a few days, these cravings tend to disappear and we may be amazed that we don't miss some of our convenience or "comfort" foods as much as we thought we would. If one has been addicted to a food like sugar for many years, it does not take much to "fall off the wagon" and be addicted again. Therefore, perseverance is the key to long-term success. As the Chinese say, a million is made up of nothing but lots of ones, and a bucket is quickly filled by steady drips and drops.

Exercise

Exercise is the second of what I call the three free therapies. According to Chinese medicine, regular, adequate exercise has two basic benefits. First, exercise promotes the movement of the qi and quickening of the blood. Since all FMS involves at least some component of qi stagnation and/or blood stasis, it is obvious that exercise is an important therapy for this condition. It helps alleviate both the stagnation causing the bodily aches and pain and the stagnation associated with liver depression. Secondly, exercise benefits the spleen and therefore treats spleen qi vacuity, the other pattern which is always involved to some degree in FMS. The spleen's movement and transportation of the digestate is dependent upon the qi mechanism. The qi mechanism describes the function of the qi in upbearing the clear and downbearing the turbid parts of digestion. For the qi mechanism to function properly, the qi must be flowing normally and freely. Since exercise moves and rectifies the qi, it also helps regulate and rectify the qi mechanism. This then results in the spleen's movement and transportation of foods and liquids and its subsequent engendering and transforming of the qi and blood. A healthy spleen produces lots of qi and lots of blood. This means that the movement of the qi is pushed and that the sinews and vessels are nourished. It also means there will be left over qi and blood to turn into yin essence to bolster and support kidney yin. Further, a healthy spleen checks and controls a depressed liver. Therefore, it is easy to see that regular, adequate exercise is a vitally important component of any regime for either preventing or treating FMS.

What kind of exercise is best for FMS?

In my experience and according to everything I have read on fibromyalgia, some combination of daily, gentle aerobic exercise and stretching is most beneficial for people with FMS. By aerobic exercise, I mean any physical activity which raises one's heartbeat 80% above their normal resting rate and keeps it there for at least 20 minutes. To calculate your normal resting heart rate, place your fingers over the pulsing artery on the front side of your neck. Count the beats for 15 seconds and then multiply by four. This gives you your beats per minute or BPM. Now multiply your BPM by 0.8. Take the resulting number and add it to your resting BPM.[2] This gives you your aerobic threshold of BPM. Next engage in any physical activity you like. After you have been exercising for five minutes, take your pulse for 15 seconds once again at the artery on the front side of your throat. Again multiply the resulting count by four and this tells you your current BPM. If this number is less than your aerobic threshold BPM, then you know you need to exercise harder or faster. Once

---

[2] Here's another method for calculating your aerobic heart rate: Take your resting pulse for six seconds and multiply by 10. Then add this number to your age. Then subtract this sum from 220, multiply by 0.6 and add your resting heart rate.

you get your heart rate up to your aerobic threshold, then you need to keep exercising at the same level of intensity for at least 20 minutes. In order to insure that one is keeping their heartbeat high enough for long enough, one should recount their pulse every five minutes or so if you have any doubt.

Depending on one's age and physical condition, different people will have to exercise harder to reach their aerobic threshold than others. For some, simply walking briskly will raise their heartbeat 80% above their resting rate. For others, they will need to do calisthenics, running, swimming, racquetball, or some other, more strenuous exercise. It really does not matter what the exercise is as long as it raises your heartbeat 80% above your resting rate and keeps it there for 20 minutes. However, there are two other criteria that should be met. One, the exercise should be something that is not too boring. If it is too boring, then you may have a hard time keeping up your schedule. Since most people do find aerobic exercises such as running, stationary bicycles, and stair-steppers boring, it is good to listen to music or watch TV in order to distract your mind from the tedium. Secondly, the type of exercise should not cause any damage to any parts of the body. For instance, running on pavement may cause knee problems for some people. Therefore, you should pick a type of exercise you enjoy but also one which will not cause any problems.

Generally, jogging, vigorous areobic dance, and weight lifting are too strenuous for most fibromyalgia patients. Because fibro-myalgia patients can so easily overexert themselves, you must be sure to start gradually and only do as much exercise per day as makes you feel better the next day. Dr. David A. Nye, an MD specializing in the treatment of fibromyalgia suggests starting with as little as 3-5 minutes of exercise and gradually working up from there.[3] According to Dr. Nye, exercise is most effective when

---

[3] Nye, David A., "A Guide for Patients with Fibromyalgia Syndrome," http://prairie.lakes.com/~roseleaf/fibro/pat-faq.html, p. 1

it is done in the late afternoon or early evening. If you absolutely can't do it then, you will probably need to exercise a bit longer earlier in the day to get the same effect. However, that doesn't mean you shouldn't exercise at all if you can't do it in the late afternoon. Dr. Nye also reminds fibromyalgia sufferers not to exercise just before bedtime as this may interfere with your sleep. If your pain is mostly in your legs and lower body, you might try doing some exercise which primarily works your arms and upper body and vice versa. Whatever kind of exercise you pick, just make sure it doesn't make you hurt worse.

Stretching is also very good for FMS. Most fibromyalgia patients say they feel tight and stiff. Stretching should be done before your aerobic exercise. This will help prevent that exercise from causing any injuries. It is also easier to stretch in the late afternoon and early evening than in the morning. Dr. Nye recommends five basic stretches for fibromyalgia sufferers. Each should be done for 20 seconds on each side. They should be gentle and painless. You will probably need to hold onto a tree or post to support yourself for stretches #4-5.

1. Shrug your shoulders in a circular motion both forward and backward one at a time, then repeat the motion with both shoulders at the same time.

2. Reach your arm over your head and bend to the opposite side.

3. Bend forward with your legs straight as if trying to touch your toes. (It doesn't matter if you can or not or how far you get. It's trying that's important.)

4. Pull your foot towards your buttock with your hand while standing on the other leg.

5. With your feet flat on the ground and one foot in front of the other, lean forward bending just the front knee. This looks like what fencers do when they lunge at their opponents.

There are many other stretches that you can do. For more ideas, check out books on yoga and stretching at your local bookstore or library. There is also a stretching video available specifically for sufferers of FMS. Its title is the *Fibromyalgia Stretch Video* and it is available from:

Oregon Fibromyalgia Foundation
1221 S.W. Yamhill, Suite 303
Portland, OR 97205

Besides aerobics, I personally try to do yoga stretches for 15-20 minutes five days per week.

Deep relaxation

As we have seen above, FMS is associated with liver depression qi stagnation. Dr. David A. Nye, quoted above, flatly says, "Stress worsens fibromyalgia."[4] In Chinese medicine, liver depression comes from not fulfilling all one's desires. But, as we have also seen above, no adult can fulfill all their desires. This is why a certain amount of liver depression is endemic among adults. When our desires are frustrated, our qi becomes depressed. This then creates emotional depression and easy anger or irritability. In Chinese medicine, anger is nothing other than the venting of pent up qi in the liver. When qi becomes depressed in the liver, it accumulates like hot air in a balloon. Eventually, that hot, depressed, angry qi has to go somewhere. So when there is a little more frustration or stress, then this angry qi in the liver may vent itself upward as irritability, anger, shouting, or nasty words. Or the accumulated qi may vent sideways to the spleen and stomach and manifest as abdominal pain, cramping, constipation or diarrhea.

Essentially, this type of anger and irritability are due to a maladaptive coping response that is typically learned at a young

---

[4] *Ibid.*, p. 5

age. When we feel frustrated or stressed, stymied by or angry about something, most of us tense our muscles and especially the muscles in our upper back and shoulders, neck, and jaws. At the same time, many of us will hold our breath. In Chinese medicine, the sinews are governed by the liver. This tensing of the muscles, *i.e.*, the sinews, constricts the flow of qi in the channels and network vessels. Since it is the liver which is responsible for the coursing and discharging of this qi, such tensing of the sinews leads to liver depression qi stagnation. Because the lungs govern the downward spreading and movement of the qi, holding our breath due to stress or frustration only worsens this tendency of the qi not to move and, therefore, to become depressed in the Chinese medical idea of the liver.

Therefore, deep relaxation is the third of the three free therapies. For deep relaxation to be therapeutic medically, it needs to be more than just mental equilibrium. It needs to be somatic or bodily relaxation as well as mental repose. Most of us no longer recognize that every thought we think and feeling we feel is actually a felt physical sensation somewhere in our body. The words we use to describe emotions are all abstract nouns, such as anger, depression, sadness, and melancholy. However, in Chinese medicine, *every emotion is associated with a change in the direction or flow of qi*. For instance, anger makes the qi move upward, while fear makes it move downward. Therefore, anger "makes our gorge rise" or "blow our top", while fear may cause a "sinking feeling" or make us "pee in our pants." These colloquial expressions are all based on the age-old wisdom that all thoughts and emotions are not just mental but also bodily events. This is why it is not just enough to clear one's mind. Clearing one's mind is good, but for really marked therapeutic results, it is even better if one clears one's mind at the same time as relaxing every muscle in the body as well as the breath.

Guided deep relaxation tapes

The single most efficient and effective way I have found for myself and my patients to practice such mental and physical deep relaxation is to do a daily, guided, progressive, deep relaxation audiotape. What I mean by guided is that a narrator on the tape leads one through the process of deep relaxation. Such tapes are progressive since they lead one through the body in a progressive manner, first relaxing one body part and then moving on to another. For instance, the narrator may say something to the effect that, as you exhale, you should feel your forehead get heavy and relaxed, softening and expanding, becoming warm and heavy. As you exhale again, now feel your cheeks get heavy and relaxed, softening and expanding, becoming warm and heavy. Breathe in and breathe out, letting your breath go without hindrance or hesitation. Breathing out, now feel your jaw muscles become heavy and relaxed, expanding and softening, becoming warm and heavy, etc., etc. throughout the entire body until one comes to the bottoms of one's feet.

There are innumerable such tapes on the market. These are usually sold in health food stores, New Age music and supply stores, or in bookstores with a good selection of New Age books. Over the years of suggesting this method of deep relaxation to my patients, I have found that each patient will have his or her own preferences in terms of the type of voice, male or female, the choice of words and imagery, whether there is background music or not, and the actual pace of the progression through the body. Therefore, I suggest listening to and even purchasing more than one such tape. One should find a tape which they like and can listen to without internal criticism or comment, going along like a cloud in the sky as the narrator's voice blows away all your mental and bodily stress and tension. If one has more than one tape, one can also switch every now and again from tape to tape so as not to become bored with the process or desensitized to the instructions.

Key things to look for in a good relaxation tape

In order to get the full therapeutic effect of such deep relaxation tapes, there are several key things to check for. First, be sure that the tape is a guided tape and not a subliminal relaxation tape. Subliminal tapes usually have music and any instructions to relax are given so quietly that they are not consciously heard. Although such tapes can help you feel relaxed when you do them, ultimately they do not teach you how to relax as a skill which can be consciously practiced and refined. Secondly, make sure the tape starts from the top of the body and works downward. Remember, anger makes the qi go upward in the body, and people with FMS due to liver depression qi stagnation already have too much qi rising upward in their bodies and becoming stagnant in their abdomens. Such depressed qi typically needs not only to be moved but also downborne. Third, make sure the tape instructs you to relax your physical body. If you do not relax all your muscles or sinews, the qi cannot flow freely and the liver cannot be coursed. Depression is not resolved, and there will not be the same medically therapeutic effect. And lastly, be sure the tape instructs you to let your breath go with each exhalation. One of the symptoms of liver depression is a stuffy feeling in the chest which we then unconsciously try to relieve by sighing. Letting each exhalation go completely helps the lungs push the qi downward. This allows the lungs to control the liver at the same time as it downbears upwardly counterflowing angry liver qi.

The importance of daily practice

When I was a medical student in Shanghai in the People's Republic of China, I was once taken on a field trip to a hospital where they were using deep relaxation as a therapy with patients with high blood pressure, heart disease, stroke, and migraines. Research at this hospital showed how such daily, progressive deep relaxation can regulate the blood pressure and body temperature and improve the appetite, digestion, elimination, sleep, energy, and mood. One of the things they said at this hospital is, "Small results in 100 days, big results in 1,000." This means that if one does such daily, progressive deep relaxation *every single day for 100 days*, one will definitely experience certain results. What are these "small" results? These small results are improvements in all the parameters listed above: blood pressure, body temperature, appetite, digestion, elimination, sleep, energy, and mood. If these are "small" results, then what are the "big" results experienced in 1,000 days of practice? The "big" results are a change in how one reacts to stress—in other words, a change in one's very personality or character.

What these doctors in Shanghai stressed and what I have also experienced both personally and with my patients is that it is vitally important to do such daily, guided, progressive deep relaxation every single day, day in and day out for a solid three months at least and for a continuous three years at best. If you do such progressive, somatic deep relaxation every day, you will see every parameter or measurement of health and well-being improve. If you do this kind of deep relaxation only sporadically, missing a day here and there, it will feel good when you do it, but it will not have the marked, cumulative therapeutic effects it can. Therefore, perseverance is the real key to getting the benefits of deep relaxation.

The real test

Doing such a daily deep relaxation regime is like hitting tennis balls against a wall or hitting a bucket of balls at a driving range. It is only practice; it is not the real game itself. A daily deep relaxation regime is done not only in order to relieve one's immediate stress and strain. It is done to learn a new skill, a new way to react to stress. The ultimate goal is to learn how to breathe out and immediately relax all one's muscles in the body in reaction to stress, rather than the common but unhealthy maladaption to stress of holding one's breath and tensing one's muscles. By doing such deep relaxation day after day, you will learn how to relax any and every muscle in your body quickly and efficiently. Then, as soon as you recognize that you are feeling frustrated, stressed out, or uptight, you can immediately remedy those feelings at the same time as coursing your liver and rectifying your qi. This is the real test, the game of life. "Small results in 100 days, big results in 1,000."

Finding the time

If you're like me and most of my patients, you are probably asking yourself right now, "All this is well and good, but when am I supposed to find the time to eat well-balanced cooked meals, exercise at least every other day, and do a deep relaxation every day? I'm already stretched to the breaking point." I know. That's the problem.

As a clinician, I often wish I could wave a magic wand over my patients' heads and make them all healthy and well. I cannot. After close to two decades of working with thousands of patients, I know of no easy way to health. There is good living and there is easy living. Or perhaps I am stating this all wrong. What most people take as the easy way these days is to continue pushing their limits continually to the max. The so-called path of least resistance is actually the path of lots and lots of resistance. Unless you take time for yourself and find the time to eat well, exercise, and relax, no treatment is going to eliminate your FMS completely. There is simply no pill you can pop or food you can eat that will get rid of the root causes of FMS: poor diet, too little exercise, and too much stress. Even Chinese herbal medicine and acupuncture can only get their full effect if the diet and lifestyle is first adjusted. Sun Si-maio, the most famous Chinese doctor of the Tang dynasty (618-907 CE), who himself refused government office and lived to be 101, said: "First adjust the diet and lifestyle and only secondarily give herbs and acupuncture." Likewise, it is said today in China, "Three parts treatment, seven parts nursing." This means that any cure is only 30% due to medical treatment and 70% is due to nursing, meaning proper diet and lifestyle.

In my experience, this is absolutely true. Seventy percent of all disease will improve after three months of proper diet, exercise, relaxation, and lifestyle modification. Seventy percent! Each of us has certain nondiscretionary rituals we perform each day. For instance, you may always and without exception find the time to brush your teeth. Perhaps it is always finding the time to shower. For others, it may be always finding the time each day to eat lunch. And for 99.99% of us, we find time, no, we make the time to get dressed each day. The same applies to good eating, exercise, and deep relaxation. Where there's a will there's a way. If your FMS is bad enough, you can find the time to eat well, get proper exercise, and do a daily deep relaxation tape.

The solution to FMS is in your hands

I live in Boulder, CO, and we have a walking mall in the center of town. On summer evenings, I and my wife often walk down this mall. Having treated so many patients over the years, it is not unusual for me to meet former patients on these strolls. Frequently, these patients begin by telling me they're sorry they haven't been in to see me in such a long time. They usually say this apologetically as if they have done something wrong. I then usually ask them how they've been. Often they tell me: "When my such-and-such flares up, I remember what you told me about my diet, exercise, and lifestyle. I then go back to doing my exercise or deep relaxation or I change my diet, and then my symptoms go away. That's why I haven't been in. I'm sorry."

However, such patients have no need to be sorry. This kind of story is music to my ears. When I hear that these patients are now able to control their own conditions by following the dietary and lifestyle advice I gave them, I know that, as a Chinese doctor, I have done my job correctly. In Chinese medicine, the inferior doctor treats disease after it has appeared. The superior doctor prevents disease before it has arisen. If I can teach my patients how to cure their symptoms themselves by making changes in their diet and lifestyle, then I'm approaching the goal of the high

115

class Chinese doctor—the prevention of disease through patient education.

To get these kinds of benefits, however, one must make the necessary changes in eating and behavior. In addition, FMS is not a condition that is cured once and forever like measles or mumps. When I say Chinese medicine can cure FMS, I do not mean that you will never experience symptoms again. What I mean is that Chinese medicine can eliminate or greatly reduce your symptoms *as long as you keep your diet and lifestyle together*. People being people, we all "fall off the wagon" from time to time and we all "choose our own poisons." I do not expect perfection from either my patients or myself. Therefore, I am not looking for a lifetime cure. Rather, I try to give my patients an understanding of what causes their disease and what they can do to minimize or eliminate its causes and mechanisms. It is then up to the patient to decide what is bearable and what is unbearable or what is an acceptable level of health. The Chinese doctor will have done their job when *you know how to correct your health to the level you find acceptable given the price you have to pay.*

12
Simple Home Remedies for FMS

Although faulty diet, lack of adequate exercise, and too much stress are the ultimate causes of FMS according to Chinese medicine and, therefore, diet, exercise, and deep relaxation are the most important in the treatment and prevention of FMS, there are a number of simple Chinese home remedies to help relieve the symptoms of fibromyalgia.

Chinese aromatherapy

In Chinese medicine, the qi is seen as a type of wind or vapor. The Chinese character for qi shows wind blowing over a rice field. In addition, smells are often referred to as a thing's qi. Therefore, there is a close relationship between smells carried through the air and the flow of qi in a person's body. Although aromatherapy has not been a major part of professionally practiced Chinese medicine for almost a thousand years, there is a simple aromatherapy treatment which one can do at home which can help alleviate irritability, depression, nervousness, anxiety, and insomnia.

In Chinese, *Chen Xiang* means "sinking fragrance." It is the name of Lignum Aquilariae Agallochae or Eaglewood. This is a frequent ingredient in Asian incense formulas. In Chinese medicine, Aquilaria is classified as a qi-rectifying medicinal. When used as a boiled decoction or "tea", Aquilaria moves the qi and stops pain, downbears upward counterflow and regulates the middle (*i.e.*, the spleen and stomach), and promotes the kidneys' grasping of the qi sent down by the lungs. I believe that the word sinking in this herb's name refers to this medicinal's downbearing of upwardly counterflowing qi. Such upwardly counterflowing qi eventually must accumulate in the heart, disturbing and causing restlessness of the heart spirit. When this medicinal wood is burnt and its smoke is inhaled as a medicinal incense, its downbearing and spirit-calming function is emphasized.

One can buy Aquilaria or *Chen Xiang* from Chinese herb stores in Chinatowns, Japantowns, or Koreatowns in major urban areas. One can also buy it from Chinese medical practitioners who have their own pharmacies. It is best to use the powdered variety. However, powder may be made by putting a small piece of this aromatic wood in a coffee grinder. It is also OK to use small bits of the wood if powder is not available. Next one needs to buy a roll of incense charcoals. Place one charcoal in a nonflammable dish and light it with a match. Then sprinkle a few pinches of Aquilaria powder on the lit charcoal. As the smoke rises, breathe in deeply. This can be done on a regular basis one or more times per day or on an as-needed basis by those suffering from restlessness, nervousness, anxiety, irritability, and depression. For those who experience insomnia, one can do this "treatment" when lying in bed at night.

This Chinese aromatherapy with Lignum Aquilariae Agallochae is very cheap and effective. I know of no side effects or contraindications.

Light therapy

Light therapy, more specifically sunbathing or heliotherapy, is one of Chinese medicine's health preservation and longevity practices. Sunlight is considered the most essential yang qi in nature. Li Shi-zhen, one of the most famous Chinese doctors of the late Ming dynasty (1368-1644 CE) wrote, "*Tai yang* (literally, supreme yang but a name for the sun) is true fire." As he pointed out, "Without fire, heaven is not able to engender things, and without fire, people are not able to live." Because the back of the human body is yang (as compared to the front which is more yin), exposing the back to sunlight is a good way of increasing one's yang qi.

As we have seen above, most people's yang qi begins to decline by around 35 years of age. In those over 35 years of age, loose stools, lack of strength, poor memory, lack of concentration, poor coordination, decline in or lack of libido, low back and knee soreness and weakness, increased nighttime urination, and cold hands and feet are mostly due to this decline first in the yang qi of the spleen and later in the yang qi of the spleen and kidneys. When some people say they are depressed, what they often mean in Chinese medical terms is that they are extremely fatigued. In such cases, sunbathing can help supplement the yang qi of the body, thereby strengthening the spleen and/or kidneys.

Furthermore, because the yang qi is also the motivating force which pushes the qi, increasing yang qi can also help resolve depression and move stagnation. Cao Ting-dong, a famous doctor of the Qing dynasty (1644-1911 CE) wrote:

> Sitting with the back exposed directly to the sun, the back may get warmed. This is able to make the entire body harmonious and smoothly flowing. The sun is the essence of *tai yang* and its light strengthens the yang qi of the human body.

In Chinese medicine, whenever the words harmonious and smoothly flowing are used together, they refer to the flow of qi and blood. Hence sunbathing can help course the liver and rectify the qi as well as fortify the spleen and invigorate the kidneys.

It has been said that sunlight is good for every disease except skin cancer. As we now know, overexposure to the sun can cause skin cancer due to sunlight damaging the cells of the skin. Therefore, one should be careful not to get too much sun and not to get burnt. In Chinese medicine, sunbathing should be done between the hours of 8-10 AM. One should only sunbathe between 11 AM-1 PM in winter in temperate, not tropical, latitudes.

119

Hydrotherapy

Hydrotherapy means water therapy and is a part of traditional Chinese medicine. There are numerous different water treatments for helping relieve various symptoms of FMS. First, let's begin with a warm bath. If one takes a warm bath just slightly higher than body temperature for 15-20 minutes, this can free and smooth the flow of qi and blood. In addition, it can calm the spirit and hasten sleep. Taking a warm bath a half hour before going to bed can help insomnia. It can also relieve tension and irritability.

However, when using a warm bath, one must be careful not to use water so hot or to stay in the bath so long that sweat breaks out on one's forehead. We lose yang qi as well as body fluids when we sweat. Because "fluids and blood share a common source", excessive sweating can cause problems for those with blood and yin vacuities. Sweating can also worsen yang qi vacuities in people whose spleen and kidneys are weak. Therefore, unless one is given a specific hot bath prescription by their Chinese medical practitioner, I suggest those with FMS not stay in warm baths until they sweat. Although they may feel pleasantly relaxed, they may later feel excessively fatigued or excessively hot and thirsty.

If, due to depression transforming heat, yang qi is exuberant and counterflowing upward, it may cause tension headaches or extreme irritability. In this case, one can tread in cold water up to their ankles for 15-20 minutes at a time. One may also soak their hands in cold water. Or they may put cold, wet compresses on the backs of their necks. The first two treatments seek to draw yang qi away from the head to either the lower part of the body or out to the extremities. The third treatment seeks to block and neutralize yang qi from counterflowing upward, congesting in the head and damaging the blood vessels in the head.

For those who are struggling with obesity, one can use cool baths slightly lower than body temperature for 10 minutes per day.

120

Although this may seem contradictory, since cold is yin and these patients already suffer from a yang insufficiency, this brief and not too extreme exposure to cool water stimulates the body to produce more yang qi. In Chinese medicine, it is not thought advisable for women to take cold baths during menstruation as this may retard the free flow of qi and blood and lead to dysmenorrhea or painful menstruation.

For abdominal pain due to qi stagnation, one can apply warm, wet compresses to the abdomen for 15-20 minutes at a time. One should not sleep with a hot water bottle or heating pad. If one uses such a hot application for too long, it begins to raise the body temperature. The body must maintain its normal temperature of 98.6° F. Therefore, if the body temperature goes up due to local application of heat, the body's response is to actually cut off the blood flow to that area of the body. This then would result in just the opposite, unwanted effect. Cooking several slices of fresh ginger in the water at a low boil for five to seven minutes and then using the resulting "tea" to make the hot compress can increase the compresses effect of moving the qi.

Chinese self-massage

Massage, including self-massage, is a highly developed part of traditional Chinese medicine. At its most basic, rubbing promotes the flow of qi and blood in the area rubbed. Below are three Chinese self-massage regimes. The first is a general protocol for mental stress that can also be used if there is insomnia, mental fatigue or poor mental concentration, the second is for diarrhea, and the third is for constipation. Crampy diarrhea or alternating with constipation is one of the key symptoms of irritable bowel syndrome, and many FMS sufferers also complain of this condition. In fact, there are Chinese self-massage regimes for many health problems such as headache, painful menstruation, nausea and vomiting, acne, all sorts of body pain, colds and flus, and dizziness. For more Chinese self-massage regimes, the reader should see Fan Ya-li's *Chinese Self-massage Therapy: The Easy Way to Health,* also published by Blue Poppy Press.

Self-massage for insomnia

Bai Hui (GV 20)

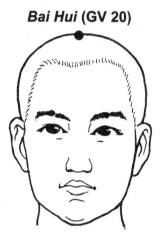

Begin by patting the top of the head with the hollow of the palm 20 times. The point in the middle of the top of the head is called *Bai Hui* (Meeting of Hundreds, Governing Vessel 20). Stimulation of this point calms the spirit and downbears upwardly counterflowing and exuberant liver yang 20 times.

Zan Zhu (BI 2)

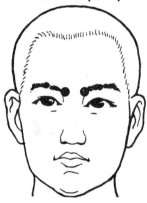

Next, use the tips of both index or middle fingers to press and knead the depression at the medial ends of the eyebrows (next to the nose) 30 times. This is the acupuncture point *Zan Zhu* (Bladder 2) which clears the head.

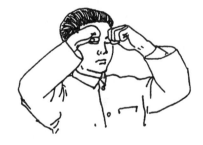

Third, bend the two index fingers and push with their radial (thumb) sides from the middle to the left and right sides of the forehead. Do this 20 times.

122

Fourth, on both sides of the head, find the spot where a line drawn horizontally half an inch above the front hairline and a line drawn vertically half an inch behind the hairline at the temple would meet. This is the point *Tou Wei* (Stomach 8). Press and knead 30 times.

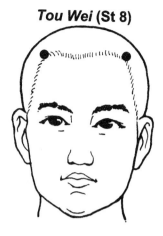

Tou Wei (St 8)

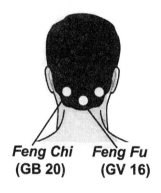

Feng Chi (GB 20) **Feng Fu (GV 16)**

Fifth, press and knead the base of the skull in the depressions on both sides of the back of the neck 30 times. This is the acupuncture point *Feng Chi* (Gallbladder 20) and is a major point for treating upwardly counter-flowing liver qi.

Sixth, press and knead the spot at the base of the skull at the midline 30 times. This point, *Feng Fu* (Governing Vessel 16), is for calming the spirit.

Seventh, press and knead *Shen Men* (Heart 7). This point is located on the inner wrist crease, just below the palm. As you are looking at your palm the point is on a line down from the little finger on the medial side of the tendon. This point also calms the spirit.

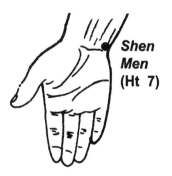

Shen Men (Ht 7)

123

Eighth, press and knead *San Yin Jiao* (Spleen 6). This point is an intersection of the spleen, liver, and kidney channels. It supplements the spleen and stomach, harmonizes the liver, and calms the spirit. It is located three inches above the tip of the inner anklebone on the back edge of the tibia or lower leg bone.

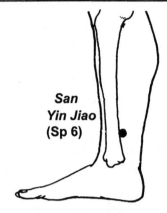

San Yin Jiao (Sp 6)

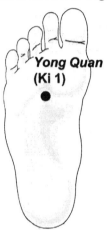

Yong Quan (Ki 1)

Finally, rub *Yong Quan* (Kidney 1) with a circular motion. This point is located on the bottom of the foot, approximately one third of the distance between the base of the second toe and the heel. *Yong Quan* supplements the kidneys, regulates the stool, calms the liver and rouses the brain.

Self-massage for chronic diarrhea

Begin by pressing and kneading four points 30 times each. First press and knead *Zhong Wan* (Conception Vessel 12). This point is located on the midline of the abdomen, halfway between the lower tip of the sternum and the navel. Next press and knead *Qi Hai* (Conception Vessel 6). This point is on the midline of the lower abdomen, two finger breadths below the navel.

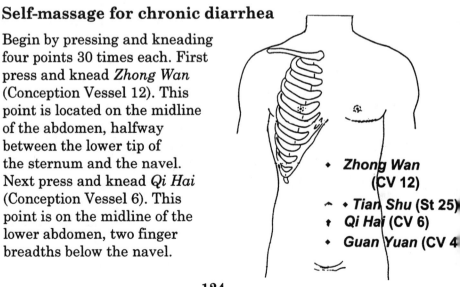

• **Zhong Wan (CV 12)**

• **Tian Shu (St 25)**

• **Qi Hai (CV 6)**

• **Guan Yuan (CV 4)**

Then press and knead *Quan Yuan* (Conception Vessel 4). This point is located four finger breadths below the navel on the midline of the lower abdomen. Finally, press and knead *Tian Shu* (Stomach 25), which is located two inches from the center of the navel on both sides.

Conception Vessel 12 regulates the spleen and stomach, the root of qi and blood engenderment and transformation. Conception Vessel 6 regulates and fortifies the qi in the entire body. Conception Vessel 4 fortifies the spleen and nourishes the kidneys. Stomach 25 regulates the spleen, stomach and intestines and is indicated for digestive symptoms including diarrhea, constipation, poor appetite, abdominal pain, and rumbling intestines.

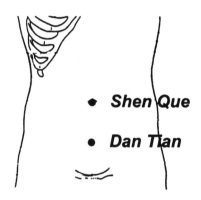

Next, use the first three fingers and rub the following two points in a counter-clockwise direction, 50 times each. *Shen Que* (Conception Vessel 8) is located at the navel. *Dan Tian* (Cinnabar Field) is located three finger breadths directly below the navel.

Third, press and knead all down the large muscles on either side of the spine. Press and knead approximately one and a half inches on either side of the spine. There are acupuncture points along the spine which connect directly with all the viscera and bowels. The production and function of the qi and blood is dependent on the proper functioning of the viscera and bowels.

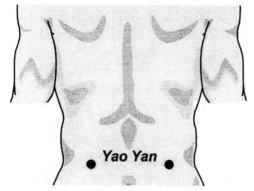

Yao Yan

Fourth, make the hand into a loose fist and use the thumb side of the hand to scrub back and forth on the point *Yao Yan* (Eyes of the Lumbus, extra point M-BW-24). *Yao Yan* is located next to the fourth lumbar ver-tebra, approximately 3.5 inches to either side.

Fifth, scrub the low back or lumbosacral region. Scrub back and forth from side to side until the area becomes warm to the touch. "The low back is the mansion of the kidneys," and this stimulates the kidneys, remembering that sufficient kidney yang is necessary for normal functioning of the spleen and stomach.

Last, press and knead three points 30 times each. The first point is *He Gu* (Large Intestine 4). Large Intestine 4 is located on the bulge of the muscle between the thumb and index finger when they are pressed together, press this point to the side against the first metacarpal bone in the hand. The second point is *Zu San Li* (Stomach 36). This point is located three inches below the lower, outside edge of the kneecap. This point regulates the qi of the entire body, regulates the qi of the stomach channel in particular, and fortifies the spleen at the same time as it harmonizes the stomach. The third point is *San Yin Jiao* (Spleen 6).

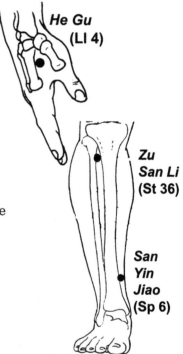

He Gu
(LI 4)

Zu
San Li
(St 36)

San
Yin
Jiao
(Sp 6)

This point is an intersection of the spleen, liver and kidney channels. It has many functions including supplementing the spleen and stomach, harmonizing the liver, nourishing the kidneys and calming the spirit. It is located three inches above the tip of the inner anklebone on the back edge of the tibia or lower leg bone.

If the diarrhea is worse with mental-emotional stress and is accompanied by abdominal pain, rumbling intestines or distention in the abdomen, ribside or chest, the following two points may be pressed and kneaded 30 times each.

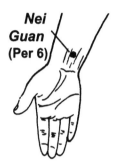

First, press and knead *Nei Guan* (Pericardium 6). This point is located on the palmar side of the forearm, two inches from the wrist crease, between the two tendons. It rectifies the qi, downbears counterflow, harmonizes the stomach and stops pain.

And finally, press and knead *Tai Chong* (Liver 3) to soothe the liver and rectify the qi. Liver 3 is on the top of the foot in the depression between the first and second metatarsal bones just distal to where the tarsal and metatarsal bones meet.

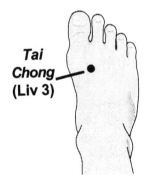

Self-massage for constipation

First, knead Stomach 25 and Conception Vessel 4, 30 times each. The locations of these points are given above in the first step of the self-massage protocol for diarrhea. Together, they fortify the spleen, nourish the kidneys and regulate the digestion.

Next, rub the lower abdomen clockwise 50 times.

Third, press and knead all down the large muscles on either side of the spine. Press and knead approximately one and a half inches on either side of the spine. There are acupuncture points along the spine which connect directly with all the viscera and bowels. The production and function of the qi and blood is dependent on the proper functioning of the viscera and bowels.

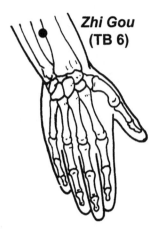

Zhi Gou (TB 6)

Fourth, press and knead *Zhi Gou* (Triple Burner 6) 30 times. This point is located on the back of the arm, three inches from the wrist between the radius and the ulna (the two bones in the forearm). It clears the triple burner, frees the bowel qi and downbears counterflow qi and fire and is often used to treat constipation and abdominal pain.

Fifth, press and knead two points 30 times each. The first point is Large Intestine 4 and the second is Stomach 36. The locations of these two points are given under the last step of the self-massage protocol for diarrhea above. In this case, Large Intestine 4 is used to free gastrointestinal downbearing. Stomach 36 regulates the qi of the entire body, regulates the qi of the stomach channel in particular, and fortifies the spleen at the same time as it harmonizes the stomach.

Sixth, with the palms of the hands pat the side of the lower leg, from the knee to the ankle, 10 times on each leg.

Finally, grasp *Cheng Shan* (Bladder 57) 10 times. Bladder 57 is located on the back of the lower leg between the two heads of the gastrocnemius muscle. Grasping means to slowly lift, squeeze and knead the muscle with the thumb and index finger. Bladder 57 harmonizes the intestines and treats constipation.

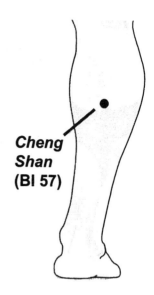

Cheng Shan (BI 57)

The key to success with Chinese self-massage therapy is perseverance. Although a single massage may provide some symptomatic relief on that very day, it is repeated self-massage day after day which can make stable and lasting changes.

Chinese foot therapy

Foot reflexology is also a part of contemporary Chinese medicine. Chinese doctors have adopted Western foot reflexology and added to it Chinese diagnosis and treatment protocols. According to foot reflexology theory, various areas on the bottoms of the feet correspond with various viscera and bowels in the body. By stimulating these areas on the feet, one can effect the function of the corresponding viscera and bowels. Usually the method of stimulation is a strong, kneading pressure on the associated areas to be treated. One can use either the ball of their thumb or the eraser on a pencil. Shops selling massage implements often have special wooden foot zone stimulators. In order to increase the circulation in the feet to make this therapy even more effective, one can soak the feet in warm or hot water prior to treatment.

Insomnia

To treat insomnia, strongly stimulate the following reflex zones on the bottoms of the feet: forehead sinuses, parathyroid, head, cerebellum, thyroid, spleen, and kidneys. Please note that, because the internal organs are not arranged symmetrically, the zones on the feet are also not bilaterally symmetrical. Treat one time per day during acute episodes and taper off as the insomnia likewise recedes in severity.

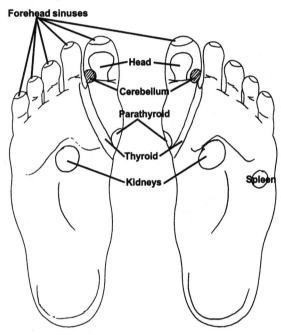

"Brain fog"

To treat poor memory, difficulty thinking and concentrating, and other similar cognitive disturbances often referred to by FMS sufferers as "brain fog," strongly stimulate the following reflex zones on the bottom of the feet: cerebellum, thyroid, adrenals, pituitary, spleen, kidneys, and heart. Please note that, because the internal organs are not arranged symmetrically, the zones on the feet are also not bilaterally symmetrical. Treat one time per day during acute episodes and taper off as the thinking becomes more clear.

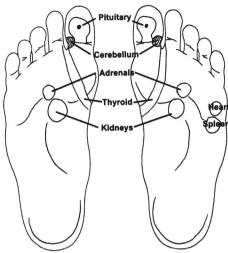

Impediment pain

To treat impediment pain, strongly stimulate the following reflex zones on the bottoms of the feet: spleen, kidneys, adrenals, lungs, upper body lymph, lower body lymph, chest area lymph, and the areas corresponding to the body parts in which there is pain. Please note that, because the internal organs are not arranged symmetrically, the zones on the feet are also not bilaterally symmetrical. Treat one time per day during acute episodes and taper off as the pain becomes less.

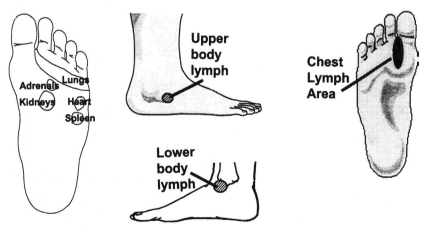

Diarrhea

To treat diarrhea, strongly stimulate the following reflex zones on the bottoms of the feet: spleen, stomach, liver, ascending, transverse, and descending colon. Please note that, because the internal organs are not arranged symmetrically, the zones on the feet are also not bilaterally symmetrical. Treat one time per day during acute episodes and taper off as the diarrhea likewise recedes in severity.

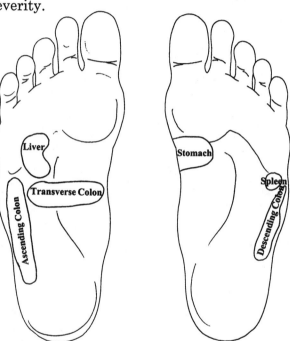

Constipation

For constipation, strongly stimulate the following foot reflex zones: rectum, anus, ascending, transverse, and descending colon. If there is liver depression qi stagnation, as there usually is in FMS, also stimulate the liver. If there is spleen vacuity, also stimulate the spleen. Treat one time per day or every other day.

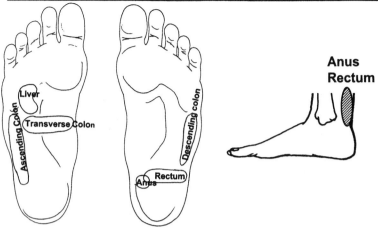

Frequent urination & incontinence

For frequent urination and incontinence as in interstitial cystitis, strongly stimulate the following foot reflex zones: kidneys, bladder, ureters, prostate (in men), urethra, and pituitary. Please note that, because the internal organs are not arranged symmetrically, the zones on the feet are also not bilaterally symmetrical. Treat one time per day during acute episodes and taper off as the frequency of urination decreases or control over bladder function increases.

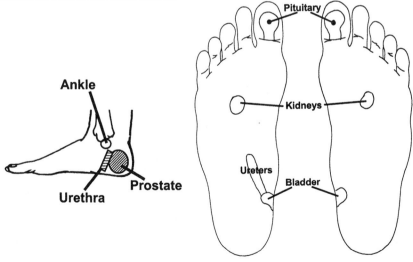

Low-grade fever

For low-grade fever, strongly stimulate the following foot reflex zones: cerebellum, pituitary, forehead sinuses, liver, kidneys, spleen, upper body lymph, lower body lymph, and chest area lymph. Please note that, because the internal organs are not arranged symmetrically, the zones on the feet are also not bilaterally symmetrical. Treat one time per day during acute episodes and taper off as the frequency of the fever decreases.

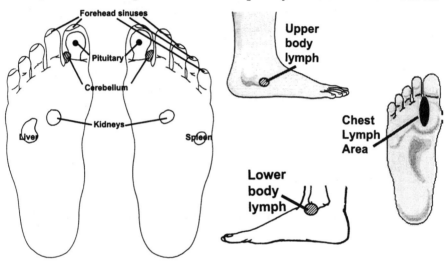

Topical application of Chinese medicinals

Another safe and simple way of stimulating the healing properties of the acupuncture points is to apply Chinese medicinals to those points. Since treating sleep disorders is such a large part of the overall treatment of fibromyalgia, having a number of different methods for improving the sleep is a good idea for this disease. The first method for treating insomnia by the external application of Chinese medicinals is to grind up 3-5 grams of Cinnabar (*Zhu Sha*) into powder. Make a paste with warm water and spread this on the point *Yong Quan* (Kidney 1) described in the above Chinese self-massage protocol. Do this on both feet. Cinnabar is one of the famous spirit-quieting medicinals of Chinese medicine. Although this medicinal's internal use is debatable, its use externally is both safe and effective. Apply this paste in the evening before bed, holding it in place with an adhesive plaster. Remove this plaster and wash off in the morning upon arising.

A second method is to grind 9 grams of Fructus Evodiae Rutecarpae (*Wu Zhu Yu*) into powder and mix into a paste with vinegar. Apply this paste over *Yong Quan* (Kidney 1) on both sides. Do this before bed each night, and then remove and wash off this paste in the morning on arising.

And a third external application is to powder some Fructus Evodiae Rutecarpae (*Wu Zhu Yu*) and Cortex Cinnamomi Cassiae (*Rou Gui*). Mix this with some warm alcohol and make into a paste. Apply this paste before bed at night to *Yong Quan* (Kidney 1) and remove in the morning. Unlike the internal Chinese herbal treatment of insomnia which typically takes three to four days to really show results, these external Chinese herbal therapies can help deepen and prolong the sleep the very first night.

Seven star hammering

A seven star hammer is a small hammer or mallet with seven small needles embedded in its head. Nowadays in China, it is often called a skin or dermal needle. It is one of the ways a person can stimulate various acupuncture points without actually inserting a needle into the body. Seven star hammers can be used either for people who are afraid of regular acupuncture, for children, or for those who wish to treat their condition at home. When the points to be stimulated are on the front of the body, this technique can be done by oneself. When they are located on the back of the body, this technique can be done by a family member or friend. This is a very easy technique which does not require any special training or expertise.

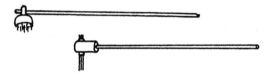

At least part of the seven star treatment for insomnia will require a helper. First, disinfect all the areas of the skin which are going to be tapped. Then begin by lightly tapping on the back of the neck. One should lightly tap all along the center of the spine on the neck as well as up and down the strap muscles to either side of the spinal column.

Then one should lightly tap acupoints *Feng Chi* (Gallbladder 20). The location of these points is behind the ear mastoid processes at the base of the skull. If one suffers from ascendant hyper-activity of liver yang, one can tap till the points bleed just a little bit. This helps drain heat or fire from the upper body. Otherwise tap until the skin is simply flushed red.

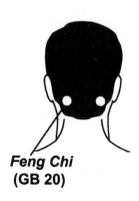

**Feng Chi
(GB 20)**

Next, tap all over the sacrum lightly until it turns a light red color. This is the triangular shaped bone at the base of the spine.

Follow this by tapping *Nei Guan* (Pericardium 6), *Shen Men* (Heart 7), and *San Yin Jiao* (Spleen 6) in that order. The locations of these three points have also been given under the section on Chinese self-massage below.

If there is headache due to ascendant hyperactivity of liver yang, tap over both temples. If the headache is severe, tap till just a little blood is let.

If there is any bleeding, wipe the area with a cotton swab moistened in alcohol or hydrogen peroxide. Then take a dry cotton ball and press the area. Between treatments, soak the seven star hammer in alcohol or hydrogen peroxide and do not share hammers between people in order to prevent any infection from one person to another. Seven star hammers are very cheap. So each person can easily afford to have their own. They can also be purchased from Oriental Medical Supply Co. whose address and phone numbers are given in the section on Chinese magnet therapy below.

Flower therapy

People have been bringing other people flowers for millennia to help them feel good. In Chinese medicine, there is actually a practice of flower therapy. Because the beauty of flowers bring most people joy and because joy is the antidote to the other four or seven negative emotions of Chinese medicine, flowers can help promote the free and easy flow of qi. It is said in Chinese medicine that, "Joy leads to relaxation (in the flow of qi)", and relaxation is exactly what the doctor ordered in cases of liver depression qi stagnation. As Wu Shi-ji wrote in the Qing dynasty, "Enjoying flowers can divert a person from their boredom and alleviate suffering caused by the seven affects (or emotions)."

However, there is more to Chinese flower therapy than the beauty of flowers bringing joy. Flower therapy also includes aromatherapy. A number of Chinese medicinals come from plants which have flowers used in bouquets. For instance,

137

Chrysanthemum flowers (*Ju Hua*, Flos Chrysanthemi Morifolii) are used to calm the liver and clear depressive heat rising to the upper body. The aroma of Chrysanthemum flowers thus also has a salutary, relaxing, and cooling effect on liver depression and depressive heat. Rose (*Mei Gui Hua*, Flos Rosae Rugosae) is used in Chinese medicine to move the qi and quicken the blood. Smelling the fragrance of Roses also does these same things. Other flowers used in Chinese medicine to calm the spirit and relieve stress and irritability are Lily, Narcissus, Lotus flowers, Orchids, and Jasmine. And further, taking a smell of a bouquet of flowers promotes deep breathing, and this, in turn, relieves pent up qi in the chest at the same time as it promotes the flow of qi downward via the lungs.

Thread moxibustion

Thread moxibustion refers to burning extremely tiny cones or "threads" of aged Oriental mugwort directly on top of certain acupuncture points. When done correctly, this is a very simple and effective way of adding yang qi to the body without causing a burn or scar.

To do thread moxa, one must first purchase the finest grade Japanese moxa wool. This is available from Oriental Medical Supply Co. mentioned below under magnet therapy. It is listed under the name Gold Direct Moxa. Pinch off a very small amount of this loose moxa wool and roll it lightly between the thumb and forefinger. What you want to wind up with is a very loose, very thin thread of moxa smaller than a grain of rice. It is important that this thread not be too large or too tightly wrapped.

Next, rub a very thin film of Tiger Balm or Temple of Heaven Balm on the point to be moxaed. These are camphorated Chinese medical salves which are widely available in North American health food stores. Be sure to apply nothing more than the thinnest film of salve. If such a Chinese medicated salve is not available, then wipe the point with a tiny amount of vegetable oil. Stand the thread of moxa up perpendicularly directly over the point to be moxaed. The oil or balm should provide enough stickiness to make the thread stand on end. Light the thread with a burning incense stick. As the thread burns down towards the skin, you will feel more and more heat. Immediately remove the burning thread when you begin to feel the burning thread go from hot to too hot. *Do not burn yourself.* It is better to pull the thread off too soon than too late. In this case, more is not better than enough. (If you do burn yourself, apply some *Ching Wan Hong* ointment. This is a Chinese burn salve which is available at Chinese apothecaries and is truly wonderful for treating all sorts of burns. It should be in every home's medicine cabinet.)

Having removed the burning thread and extinguished it between your two fingers, repeat this process again. To make this process go faster and more efficiently, one can roll a number of threads before starting the treatment. Each time the thread burns down close to the skin, pinch it off the skin and extinguish it *before* it starts to burn you. If you do this correctly, your skin will get red and hot to the touch but you will not raise a blister. Because everyone's skin is different, the first time you do this, only start out with three or four threads. Each day, increase this number until you reach nine to twelve threads per treatment.

This treatment is especially effective for women in their late 30s and throughout their 40s and men over 50 whose spleen and kidney yang qi has already become weak and insufficient. Since this treatment actually adds yang qi to the body, this type of thread moxa fortifies the spleen and invigorates the kidneys, warming yang and boosting the qi. Because the stimuli is not that strong at any given treatment, it must be done every day for a number of days. For people who suffer from FMS with pronounced fatigue, loose stools, cold hands and feet, low or no libido, and low back or knee pain accompanied by frequent nighttime urination which tends to be copious and clear, I recommend that this moxibustion be done every day for a month, stopped for a week or so, and then repeated. It can be done for several months in a row, but should not usually be done continuously throughout the year, day in and day out. Whenever symptoms get better it means that the treatment is no longer needed and should be stopped.

There are three points which should be moxaed using this supplementing technique. These are:

Qi Hai (Conception Vessel 6)
Guan Yuan (Conception Vessel 4)
Zu San Li (Stomach 36)

We have already discussed how to locate these three points above. However, I recommend visiting a local professional acupuncturist so that they can teach you how to do this technique safely and effectively and to show you how to locate these three points accurately.

In Chinese medicine, this technique is considered a longevity and health preservation technique. It is great for those people whose yang qi has already begun to decline due to the inevitable aging process. It should not be done by people with ascension of hyperactive liver yang, liver fire, or depressive liver heat. It should also always be done starting from the topmost point and moving downward. This is to prevent leading heat to counterflow upward. If there is any doubt about whether this technique is appropriate for you, please see a professional practitioner for a diagnosis and individualized recommendation.

Magnet therapy

Magnet therapy means the treatment of various regions of the body by various sized and strengths of magnets. Although magnet therapy is currently experiencing something of a vogue here in the West, magnet therapy has been a part of traditional Chinese medicine since at least the Tang dynasty. Various sized self-adhesive magnets can be purchased from:

Oriental Medical Supplies Co. (OMS)
1950 Washington St.
Braintree, MA
Tel: 1-617-331-3370 or 800-323-1839
Fax: 1-617-335-5779

For the treatments given below, I recommend using 400-800 gauss magnets. Gauss means the strength of the magnets. The ones OMS sells range in strength from 400-9,000 gauss.

Insomnia

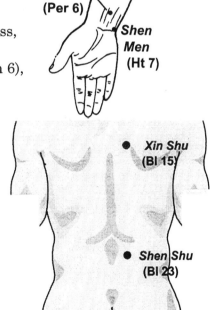

For insomnia, heart palpitations, anxiety, agitation, and restlessness, choose from among *Shen Men* (Heart 7), *Nei Guan* (Pericardium 6), *Xin Shu* (Bladder 15), *Zu San Li* (Stomach 36), and *Shen Shu* (Bladder 23).

Heart 7 and Pericardium 6 both quiet the spirit and promote sound sleep. Heart 7 is located at the medial or ulnar end of the transverse crease of the wrist in the depression just medial or inside the tendon at the side of the wrist.

Pericardium 6 is located two inches above the transverse crease of the wrist between the two tendons in the middle of the forearm.

Bladder 15 is the back transport point of the heart and has a direct connection to that organ. It is located one and a half inches lateral to the lower border of the spinous process 5th thoracic vertebra.

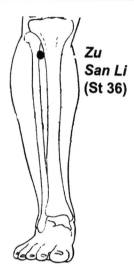

Stomach 36 fortifies the spleen and boosts the qi. It is located three inches below the outside or lateral eye of the knee and one finger's breadth lateral to the lateral edge of the tibia.

Bladder 23 is the back transport point of the kidneys. It is located one and a half inches lateral to the lower border of the spinous process of the 2nd lumbar vertebra. See illustration at the bottom of page 141.

In case of dizziness, add *Zhi Yin* (Bladder 67). It is located on the outside or lateral edge of the small toe, one tenth of an inch from the corner of the nail bed.

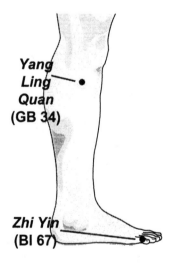

In case of liver depression qi stagnation, add *Yang Ling Quan* (Gallbladder 34). Depression of the liver qi usually exhibits oppression and distention of the rib-side, acid regurgitation, and irritability. It is located in the depression just below and slightly in front of the head of the fibula on the lower leg.

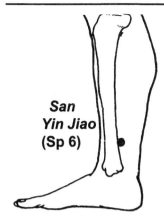

San Yin Jiao (Sp 6)

In case of liver-kidney vacuity, add *San Yin Jiao* (Spleen 6). Kidney vacuity is often manifested by frequent nighttime urination, low back weakness and/or aching, weak knees, and aversion to cold. It is located four fingers width above the tip of the inside or medial anklebone just behind the rear edge of the tibia.

Use 3-5 points each time, adhering the magnets with the south pole in touch with the skin in case of repletion and with the north pole in touch with the skin in case of vacuity. Generally, all of these points should be stimulated with the north side touching the skin in cases of fibromyalgia except Pericardium 6 and Gallbladder 34 which should be stimulated with the south side of the magnet in contact with the surface of the skin. Use small magnets on all these points.

Diarrhea & intestinal cramps

For diarrhea and intestinal cramps, choose from among *Zhong Wan* (Conception Vessel 12), *Shen Que* (Conception Vessel 8, the navel), *Tian Shu* (Stomach 25), *Zu San Li* (Stomach 36), *Da Chang Shu* (Bladder 25), and *Qi Hai* (Conception Vessel 6). The locations of all these points have been discussed above. Use 3-5 of these points each treatment, adhering the magnets with the south pole in touch with the skin. It is usually the south side of adhesive magnets that is already side up. Use small-sized magnets on all these points except for Conception Vessel 12 and Conception Vessel 8 which typically require large or medium-sized ones. Leave in place for several hours to a couple of days depending on the severity of the condition and the degree of relief obtained.

For diarrhea due to more pronounced spleen qi vacuity with marked fatigue and dizziness standing up, choose instead from: *Bai Hui* (Governing Vessel 20), *Qi Hai* (Conception Vessel 6), *Guan Yuan* (Conception Vessel 4), *Wei Shu* (Bladder 21), *Zu San Li* (Stomach 36), and *Zhong Wan* (Conception Vessel 12). Use 3-5 points per treatment and make sure the north side of the magnet is face down on the skin.

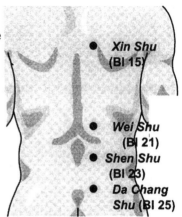

Constipation

For constipation due to either liver depression qi stagnation or heat in the stomach and intestines causing dry, hard, bound stools, choose from among *Zhong Wan* (Conception Vessel 12), *Tian Shu* (Stomach 25), *Zu San Li* (Stomach 36), *Qu Chi* (Large Intestine 11), and *Nei Ting* (Stomach 44), adhering the magnets with the south pole touching the skin. Use 3-5 points per treatment and leave in place for 2-3 days at a time. Large Intestine 11 is located at the end of the crease on the side of the elbow when it is flexed.

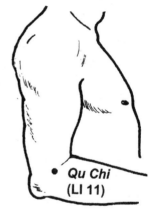

Stomach 44 is located at the end of the crease between the second and third toes on the top of the foot.

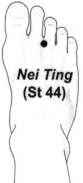

You can also use magnets locally on points of pain or on any of the 18 tender points of fibromyalgia which are indeed tender on you. Begin by trying the south side of the magnet down on top of the skin directly over the most painful spots. If that seems to aggravate the pain or doesn't improve it, try switching to the north side down. Definitely use south side down if the pain is very severe or if its nature is sharp and stabbing. For more instructions on how you might incorporate magnet therapy into your self-care, see your local acupuncturist.

Chinese herbal teas

Although some people call professionally prescribed Chinese medicinal decoctions Chinese herbal teas, this name rightly belongs to simpler, one, two, and three ingredient teas which are either steeped or boiled. Typically, such Chinese medicinal teas can be drunk throughout the day as a background beverage and can greatly enhance the effects of acupuncture and other Chinese medicinal treatment with pills and powders. The ingredients in these teas can be purchased either at Oriental specialty food stores, your local Chinese medical practitioner, from Mayway Corp. and Nuherbs Co. listed in the chapter on Chinese herbal medicine, or from:

China Herb Co.
6333 Wayne Ave.
Philadelphia, PA 19144 USA
Tel: 1-215-843-5864 / 800-221-4372
Fax: 1-215-849-3338

Impediment pain

Chinese quince tea (*Mu Gua Cha*)

This tea is made by boiling 15-20 grams of Fructus Chaenomelis Lagenariae (*Mu Gua*), 12 grams of Cortex Radicis Acanthopanacis Gracilistylis (*Wu Jia Pi*), and 6 grams of mix-fried Radix Glycyrrhizae (*Zhi Gan Cao*) in one quart of water for 15 minutes. Then strain the dregs and reserve the resulting

145

liquid for drinking during the day. It treats wind damp impediment with a simultaneous qi and blood vacuity as is common in fibromyalgia.

Sophora & Walnut Tea (*Huai Tao Cha*)

Take 15 grams each of Fructus Immaturus Sophorae Japonicae (*Huai Hua Mi*), walnuts, sesame seeds, and tea. Boil in two bowls of water till one bowl remains. Strain the dregs and drink warm. This tea treats damp heat impediment with liver-kidney vacuity and malnourishment of the sinews.

Job's tears barley & ledebouriella tea (*Yi Mi Fang Feng Cha*)

Boil 30 grams of Semen Coicis Lachryma-jobi (*Yi Yi Ren*) and 10 grams of Radix Ledebouriellae Divaricatae (*Fang Feng*) in a suitable amount of water. Strain the dregs and reserve the liquid. Use one packet per day and drink freely as tea. This tea is for wind damp impediment pain with spleen vacuity and even some liver depression.

Blood stasis pain

Rose flower tea (*Mei Gui Hua Cha*)

In Chinese medicine, rose flowers are believed to quicken the blood and dispel stasis. For either body pain associated with blood stasis or blood stasis dysmenorrhea, one can take several pieces of Flos Rosae Rugosae (*Mei Gui Hua*) and steep them along with green or black tea leaves in boiling water and then drink throughout the day as a beverage tea. Flos Rosae Rugosae, Chinese rosebuds, can be purchased from Chinese apothecaries and Chinese herbal suppliers. However, one can also use domestic rose petals or buds picked in your own garden.

Insomnia

Mulberry tea (*Sang Shen Cha*)

Boil 15 grams of Fructus Mori Albi (*Sang Shen*) in water, remove the dregs, and drink the resulting tea after dinner and before bed. It supplements the kidneys and enriches yin. It is not a sedative in the same way Western drugs are and, therefore, does not work the first night. It takes a few days for the yin to build back up again. So perseverance is required with this tea.

Abdominal cramping & pain

Hyacinth bean tea (*Bian Dou Cha*)

This tea is suitable for damp heat in the stomach and intestines causing colicky pain which comes and goes and which may be associated with either diarrhea or constipation. This tea moves the qi and transforms dampness, clears heat and drains fire. It is made by pounding 30 fresh Semen Dolichoris Lablab (*Bai Bian Dou*) or hyacinth beans into a liquid. Place in a pot, add water, and bring to a boil. Drink frequently throughout the day as a tea.

Leechee nut tea (*Li Zhi He Cha*)

This tea is suitable for liver depression qi stagnation lower abdominal pain. It is made by placing 15 grams of Semen Litchi Chinensis (*Li Zhi He*) and 10 grams of Semen Citri Reticulatae (*Ju He*) in a pot of water. Semen Citri Reticulatae are simply orange pits. Boil for 15 minutes at a medium heat. Then strain the liquid and drink freely as a tea.

Diarrhea

Plantain seed tea (*Che Qian Zi Cha*)

Stir-fry in a dry wok 10 grams of Semen Plantaginis (*Che Qian Zi*). Then steep these in boiling water with three grams of black tea. This tea is for spleen vacuity diarrhea complicated by

147

dampness. Since spleen vacuity complicates most cases of IBS, this is generally a safe tea for most IBS sufferers to drink. It even helps against damp heat diarrhea. The above prescription is for one packet or dose, and you can drink this tea 2-3 times per day as long as you are not negatively effected by black tea.

Umeboshi & kudzu tea (*Wu Mei Ge Gen Cha*)

Place one fermented plum (called umeboshi in Japanese and *Wu Mei* in Chinese) and a teaspoon of kudzu or arrowroot powder in a cup of boiling water and stir till the kudzu powder is as dissolved as possible. One can also add a slice of fresh ginger to this if you want. That makes its ability to harmonize the qi and transform dampness stronger. Drink this tea several times per day. It is very effective for stopping diarrhea.

Treating dysentery rapidly & effectively tea (*Zhi Li Su Xiao Cha*)

This tea can treat damp heat, food stagnation, and qi stagnation types of diarrhea. It is made by first stir-frying nine grams of green tea leaves in a little salt water. When the leaves are dry, combine them with nine grams of Semen Arecae Catechu (*Bin Lang*) and water in a pot. Bring to a boil and allow to steep for 10 minutes. Drink this recipe warm 2-3 times per day.

Constipation

Senna leaf tea (*Fan Xie Ye Cha*)

Senna leaves are used in Chinese medicine just the same as in Western herbalism. For heat in the stomach and intestines causing dry, hard, bound stools, steep 1-3 grams of senna leaves in boiling water. Drink this frequently as a tea.

Contraindications: Senna is a purgative and has strong laxative action that may cause abdominal pain if the dose is too strong or it is not truly appropriate. It is contraindicated during pregnancy, for nursing mothers, during menstruation, and in individuals who are vacuous and weak. It is also not suitable for long-term use.

Sesame oil & honey tea (*Xiang Mi Cha*)

This tea is for dry stools constipation due to blood vacuity and large intestine fluid dryness. Add 65 grams of honey to 35 milliliters of roasted sesame oil. Roasted sesame oil can be found in the Oriental food section of most large Western grocery food stores. Pour this mixture into boiling water and stir. Take once in the morning and once in the evening.

Biota seed & honey tea (*Bai Ren Mi Cha*)

This tea is also for dry stools constipation due to blood and fluid vacuity. Grind 15 grams of Semen Biotae Orientalis (*Bai Zi Ren*) and boil with water, Then add honey to taste and drink 1-2 times per day. This tea moistens the intestines and frees the flow of the stools, quiets the heart and aids sleep. It is indicated for habitual constipation, typically in the elderly, accompanied by heart palpitations and/or insomnia due to yin vacuity and fluid dryness.

For more information on Chinese medicinal teas, see *Chinese Medicinal Teas: Simple, Proven, Folk Formulas for Common Diseases & Promoting Health* by Zong Xiao-fang and Gary Liscum, available from Blue Poppy Press.

Chinese herbal porridges

Sometimes referred to as congee, there is a long history in Chinese medicine of combining one or two herbs with various types of porridge for the treatment and prevention of disease. There are literally hundreds of such medicinal porridge recipes in the Chinese medical literature. Chinese herbal porridges are especially useful for the treatment of all types of diarrhea and constipation. The ingredients for these porridges can be obtained from the same sources and suppliers as the Chinese herbal teas discussed above.

Insomnia

Zizyphus spinosa porridge (*Suan Zao Ren Zhou*)

This porridge is good for insomnia due to liver blood-heart yin vacuity. Stir-fry 15 grams of Semen Zizyphi Spinosae (*Suan Zao Ren*) till yellow in a dry wok or frying pain and then grind into powder. Then cook 100 grams of rice in four or five times as much water into a thin gruel. Just before the cooking is finished, stir in the powdered Zizyphus and eat on an empty stomach.

Biota seed porridge (*Bai Zi Ren Zhou*)

This porridge is also for liver-heart vacuity insomnia. Pound 15 grams of Semen Biotae Orientalis (*Bai Zi Ren*). Add to 60 grams of rice and cook into a thin gruel with plenty of water. Eat two times per day in the morning and evening. It will take two to three days before the effects of these two porridges will be felt.

Albizzia flower porridge (*He Huan Hua Zhou*)

This porridge nourishes heart blood as well as rectifies the qi of the liver and quickens the blood. It is made by first cooking 50g of rice into porridge. At the end of the cooking, stir in 30g of Flos Albizziae Julibrissin (*He Huan Hua*). Eat warm on an empty stomach one hour before going to bed each evening. This porridge is a little faster acting and is especially good when there is more pronounced liver depression and emotional tension.

Breast distention & pain

Green orange peel porridge (*Qing Pi Zhou*)

This porridge is for liver depression qi stagnation resulting in premenstrual breast distention and pain. First boil 10 grams of Pericarpium Citri Reticulatae Viride (*Qing Pi*) in a couple of cups of water for 30 minutes. Then add the resulting liquid to 50 grams of rice and more water. Cook this into porridge and eat warm two times per day beginning each month at the first signs of breast distention and pain.

Diarrhea

Kudzu & rice porridge (*Ge Gen Fen Zhou*)

This porridge is good for spleen vacuity and damp heat types of diarrhea. It is also good for tight shoulders and neck. It is made by cooking 30 grams of powdered kudzu or arrowroot with 50 grams of rice in a quart of water for several hours at a low boil. Once cooked, it can be eaten warm several times per day.

Chinese yam & egg yolk porridge (*Shan Yao Ji Zi Zhou*)

This porridge is for enduring diarrhea of many days duration due primarily to spleen vacuity. It also treats dual spleen and kidney vacuity, the two most commonly vacuous and insufficient viscera in fibromyalgia. It is made by first powdering 50 grams of Radix Dioscoreae Oppositae (*Shan Yao*). Add water to form a thin gruel and bring to a boil 2-3 times. Then add and stir in the egg yolks. Eat this three times per day on an empty stomach.

Chinese yam & plantain seed porridge (*Shan Yao Che Qian Zi Zhou*)

Powder 30 grams of Radix Dioscoreae Oppositae (*Shan Yao*), add water, and stir into a thin gruel. Then add 12 grams of Semen Plantaginis (*Che Qian Zi*) wrapped in cheesecloth or a small cotton bag. Cook the resulting mixture into porridge and eat several times per day. It treats spleen vacuity with dampness and even some damp heat.

Cardamon porridge (*Bai Dou Kou Zhou*)

This porridge is for liver-spleen disharmony diarrhea with dampness. To make it, first cook 50 grams of rice in a quart of water into a thin porridge or gruel. During the last five minutes of cooking, add five grams of powdered cardamon. Eat this three times per day (along with other foods).

Constipation

Prune seed porridge (*Yu Li Ren Zhou*)

Soak five grams of prune seeds and remove the skins. Then mash into a paste. Cook 50 grams of rice into porridge with a quart of water. Then add the mashed prune seeds, a suitable amount of honey, and a little ginger juice. Eat on an empty stomach. This porridge is for the treatment of both qi stagnation and intestinal dryness constipation due to blood and/or yin vacuity.

Pine nut porridge (*Song Ren Zhou*)

Cook 50 grams of rice and 30 grams of pine nuts in one quart of water into porridge. Add a suitable amount of honey at the end and eat two times per day on an empty stomach. This porridge treats fluid dryness constipation with hard, dry, bound stools often associated with blood and/or yin vacuity.

For numerous other Chinese herbal porridge recipes, see my *The Book of Jook: Chinese Medicinal Porridges, A Healthy Alternative to the Typical Western Breakfast* also available from Blue Poppy Press.

Obviously not every fibromyalgia sufferer will want or even need to use all the home remedies suggested in this chapter. I have given a large number of home remedies in the hopes that everyone with fibromyalgia will be able to find the materials and ingredients for at least a couple of these. Chinese medicine "makes haste slowly." So I recommend picking one or two or three of these home remedies and then sticking with them on a daily basis for some time. Daily perseverance is especially important with treatments like seven star hammer, self-massage, and foot reflexology. As an example of one possible selection from the above remedies, one might select one of the physical therapies, *i.e.*, self-massage, magnet therapy, or seven star hammer, and then combine this with a suitable Chinese herbal tea and a Chinese herbal porridge. If there was severe insomnia, one could also add one of the topical applications of Chinese medicinals for treatment of restless sleep during the night itself. The point is that A) you do not have to do everything suggested in this chapter, and B) you should persevere on a daily basis with the treatments you do choose.

13
Chinese Medical Research on Fibromyalgia

Fibromyalgia is not yet a disease diagnosis in the People's Republic of China where the overwhelming majority of research is carried out on acupuncture and Chinese medicine. Since the early 1980s, there are reams of published research on acupuncture and Chinese medicine in terms of insomnia, muscle-joint pain, fatigue, depression, fibrocystic breast disease, headaches, allergies, dysmenorrhea, and PMS, just to name some of the most common manifestations of FMS. For examples of this Chinese medical research, please see Blue Poppy Press's other *Curing* books which typically do include a chapter of abstracts of recently published Chinese research on the particular disease associated with each title. Because Chinese physicians typically do adopt Western disease names and diagnoses, I feel confident that the Chinese will soon be publishing articles on fibromyalgia. For instance, this was the first year (1999) I found the disease "chronic fatigue syndrome" discussed in a research article in a Chinese medical journal. Given the fast pace of Westernization in China, with all its attendant stress and dietary changes, can fibromyalgia be far behind?

However, there are two recently published pieces of Western research on acupuncture and fibromylagia. The first is authored by B. M. Berman, J. Ezzo, V. Hadhazy, and J. P. Swyers. It is titled *"Is Acupuncture Effective in the Treatment of Fibromyalgia."* This article was published in the March 1999 issue of

The Journal of Family Practice.[1] This study was a literature review that looked at seven other published studies on acupuncture and fibromyalgia. Three of these seven were randomized, prospective, controlled trials, while the other four were retrospective cohort studies or clinical audits. Prospective trials mean the researchers enrolled a group of fibromyalgia patients to test a specific treatment or hypothesis. A retrospective clinical audit merely looks back on the treatment of fibromyalgia patients who all received the same or similar treatment.[2] The conclusion of the authors of this literary review is that real acupuncture based on Oriental theories and techniques is more effective for the treatment of fibromyalgia than merely sticking needles in people at random locations. In other words, there is something scientifically provable about the efficacy of acupuncture for FMS.

The second study is even more positive. It was written by H. Sprott, S. Frank, and G. Hein and is titled "Pain Treatment of Fibromyalgia by Acupuncture." It appeared in 1998 in the journal, *Rheumatology International.*[3] In this study, 29 FMS patients were treated with acupuncture. Twenty-five of these were women and four were men. Their median age was 48.2 years plus or minus two years. The mean duration of their disease was 6.1 years plus or minus one year. During this study, no other medication or treatment was allowed. The severity of these patients' pain was assessed at the beginning of this study as was the number of 18 FMS tender points. In addition, serotonin levels were measured in the platelets and in the blood serum.

---

[1] *Op. cit.*, p. 213-218

[2] Clinical audits are the most common kind of Chinese medical research done in the People's Republic of China. Therefore, these four studies may actually have been Chinese studies that I missed. There are more than 30 traditional Chinese medical journals published 12 times per year in the PRC and each typically carries 30-40 articles per issue.

[3] *Op. cit.*, 18:1, p. 35-36

The patients all underwent a course of acupuncture therapy and were measured and assessed again. What this study showed was that the severity of these patients' fibromylagia definitely decreased after receiving acupuncture. In addition, less tender points were painful to pressure, their serotonin concentrations in their platelets decreased, and their serum serotonin increased. Thus this study also confirms that acupuncture does help FMS sufferers in terms of their muscle-joint pain.

Here in the West, most professional practitioners of Chinese medicine practice both acupuncture and Chinese herbal medicine. My expectation is that, in the future, research of this combined approach will be done and, when it is done, the results will be even more positive than the above trials of acupuncture alone. Because so many FMS patients have qi and yin vacuities which tend to respond better to Chinese herbal medicine, while impediment conditions and static blood do respond well to acupuncture, in my experience, the coordination of these two treatment modalities is better than either one alone.

14
Finding a Professional Practitioner of Chinese Medicine & FMS Support

Traditional Chinese medicine is one of the fastest growing holistic health care systems in the West today. At the present time, there are 50 colleges in the United States alone which offer 3-4 year training programs in acupuncture, moxibustion, Chinese herbal medicine, and Chinese medical massage. In addition, many of the graduates of these programs have done postgraduate studies at colleges and hospitals in China, Taiwan, Hong Kong, and Japan. Further, a growing number of trained Oriental medical practitioners have immigrated from China, Japan, and Korea to practice acupuncture and Chinese herbal medicine in the West.

Traditional Chinese medicine, including acupuncture, is a discreet and independent health care profession. It is not simply a technique that can easily be added to the array of techniques of some other health care profession. The study of Chinese medicine, acupuncture, and Chinese herbs is as rigorous as is the study of allopathic, chiropractic, naturopathic, or homeopathic medicine. Previous training in any one of these other systems does not automatically confer competence or knowledge in Chinese medicine. In order to get the full benefits and safety of Chinese medicine, one should seek out professionally trained and credentialed practitioners.

In the United States of America, recognition that acupuncture and Chinese medicine are their own independent professions has led to the creation of the National Commission for the Certification of Acupuncture & Oriental Medicine (NCCAOM). This commission has created and administers a national board examination in both acupuncture and Chinese herbal medicine in order to insure minimum levels of professional competence and safety. Those who pass the acupuncture exam append the letters Dipl. Ac. (Diplomate of Acupuncture) after their names, while those who pass the Chinese herbal exam use the letters Dipl. C.H. (Diplomate of Chinese Herbs). I recommend that persons wishing to experience the benefits of acupuncture and Chinese medicine should seek treatment in the U.S. only from those who are NCCAOM certified.

In addition, in the United States, acupuncture is a legal, independent health care profession in more than half the states. A few other states require acupuncturists to work under the supervision of MDs, while in a number of states, acupuncture has yet to receive legal status. In states where acupuncture is licensed and regulated, the names of acupuncture practitioners can be found in the *Yellow Pages* of your local phone book or through contacting your State Department of Health, Board of Medical Examiners, or Department of Regulatory Agencies. In states without licensure, it is doubly important to seek treatment only from NCCAOM diplomates.

When seeking a qualified and knowledgeable practitioner, word of mouth referrals are important. Satisfied patients are the most reliable credential a practitioner can have. It is appropriate to ask the practitioner for references from previous patients treated for the same problem. It is best to work with a practitioner who communicates effectively enough for the patient to feel understood and for the Chinese medical diagnosis and treatment plan to make sense. In all cases, a professional practitioner of Chinese medicine should be able and willing to give a written traditional Chinese diagnosis of the patient's pattern upon request.

For further information regarding the practice of Chinese medicine and acupuncture in the United States and for referrals to local professional associations and practitioners in the United States, prospective patients may contact:

National Commission for the Certification of Acupuncture & Oriental Medicine
P.O. Box 97075
Washington DC 20090-7075
Tel: (202) 232-1404
Fax: (202) 462-6157

The National Acupuncture & Oriental Medicine Alliance
14637 Starr Rd, SE
Olalla, WA 98357
Tel: (206) 851-6895
Fax: (206) 728-4841
e-mail: 76143.2061@compuserve.com

The American Association of Oriental Medicine
433 Front St.
Catasauqua, PA 18032-2506
Tel: (610) 433-2448
Fax: (610) 433-1832

One can also find referrals to local professional practitioners of acupuncture and Chinese medicine in the U.S. at the following Web sites:

www.acupuncture.com
www.craneherb.com
www.redwingbooks.com

Finding FMS Support

FMS is a chronic, debilitating, stressful disease, and there are four large national organizations providing support for FMS sufferers. These are:

Fibromyalgia Alliance of America, Inc.
P.O. Box 21990
Columbus, OH 43221-0990
Tel: (614)-457-4222
Fax: (614)-457-2729

Fibromyalgia Network
P.O. Box 31750
Tucson, AZ 85751-1750
Tel: 520-290-5508 or 800-853-2929
Fax: 520-290-5550

USA Fibromyalgia Association
P.O. Box 1483
Dublin, OH
Tel: 614-851-9177

National Fibromyalgia Research Association
P.O. Box 500
Salem, OR 97308

15
Learning More About Chinese Medicine

For more information on Chinese medicine in general, see:

The Web That Has No Weaver: Understanding Chinese Medicine by Ted Kaptchuk, Congdon & Weed, NY, 1983. This is the best overall introduction to Chinese medicine for the serious lay reader. It has been a standard since it was first published over a dozen years ago and it has yet to be replaced.

Chinese Secrets of Health & Longevity by Bob Flaws, Sound True, Boulder, CO, 1996. This is a six tape audiocassette course introducing Chinese medicine to lay people. It covers basic Chinese medical theory, Chinese dietary therapy, Chinese herbal medicine, acupuncture, *qi gong*, *feng shui*, deep relaxation, lifestyle, and more.

Fundamentals of Chinese Medicine by the East Asian Medical Studies Society, Paradigm Publications, Brookline, MA, 1985. This is a more technical introduction and overview of Chinese medicine intended for professional entry level students.

Traditional Medicine in Contemporary China by Nathan Sivin, Center for Chinese Studies, University of Michigan, Ann Arbor, 1987. This book discusses the development of Chinese medicine in China in the last half century as well as introducing all the basic concepts of Chinese medical theory and practice.

Rooted in Spirit: The Heart of Chinese Medicine by Claude Larre & Elisabeth Rochat de la Vallée, trans. by Sarah Stang, Station Hill Press, NY, 1995. This book explains the central concepts of Chinese medicine from a decidedly spiritual point of view. Essentially, it is commentary on the eight chapters of the *Nei Jing Ling Shu (Inner Classic: Spiritual Pivot)*.

In the Footsteps of the Yellow Emperor: Tracing the History of Traditional Acupuncture by Peter Eckman, Cypress Book Company, San Francisco, 1996. This book is a history of Chinese medicine and especially acupuncture. In it, the author traces how acupuncture came to Europe and America from China, Hong Kong, Taiwan, Japan, and Korea in the early and middle part of this century. Included are nontechnical discussions of basic Chinese medical theory and concepts.

Knowing Practice: The Clinical Encounter of Chinese Medicine by Judith Farquhar, Westview Press, Boulder, CO, 1994. This book is a more scholarly approach to the recent history of Chinese medicine in the People's Republic of China as well as an introduction to the basic methodology of Chinese medical practice. Although written by an academic sinologist and not a practitioner, it nonetheless contains many insightful and perceptive observations on the differences between traditional Chinese and modern Western medicines.

Imperial Secrets of Health and Longevity by Bob Flaws, Blue Poppy Press, Boulder, CO, 1994. This book includes a section on Chinese dietary therapy and generally introduces the basic concepts of good health according to Chinese medicine.

Chinese Herbal Remedies by Albert Y. Leung, Universe Books, NY, 1984. This book is about simple Chinese herbal home remedies.

Legendary Chinese Healing Herbs by Henry C. Lu, Sterling Publishing, Inc., NY, 1991. This book is a fun way to begin learning about Chinese herbal medicine. It is full of interesting and entertaining anecdotes about Chinese medicinal herbs.

The Mystery of Longevity by Liu Zheng-cai, Foreign Languages Press, Beijing, 1990. This book is also about general principles and practice promoting good health according to Chinese medicine.

For more information on Chinese dietary therapy, see:

The Tao of Healthy Eating According to Traditional Chinese Medicine by Bob Flaws, Blue Poppy Press, Boulder, CO, 1997. This book is a laypersons primer on Chinese dietary therapy. It includes detailed sections on the clear, bland diet as well as sections on chronic candidiasis and allergies. It also includes the Chinese medical descriptions and uses of 200 commonly eaten foods.

The Book of Jook: Chinese Medicinal Porridges, A Healthy Alternative to the Typical Western Breakfast by Bob Flaws, Blue Poppy Press, Boulder, CO, 1995. This book is specifically about Chinese medicinal porridges made with very simple combinations of Chinese medicinal herbs.

The Tao of Nutrition by Maoshing Ni, Union of Tao and Man, Santa Monica, CA 1989

Harmony Rules: The Chinese Way of Health Through Food by Gary Butt & Frena Bloomfield, Samuel Weiser, Inc., York Beach, ME, 1985

Chinese System of Food Cures: Prevention & Remedies by Henry C. Lu, Sterling Publishing Inc., NY, 1986

A Practical English-Chinese Library of Traditional Chinese Medicine: Chinese Medicated Diet ed. by Zhang En-qin, Shanghai College of Traditional Chinese Medicine Publishing House, Shanghai, 1990

Eating Your Way to Health—Dietotherapy in Traditional Chinese Medicine by Cai Jing-feng, Foreign Languages Press, Beijing, 1988

For more information on Chinese medicine and insomnia, depression, headaches, irritable bowel syndrome, PMS, fibrocystic breast disease, arthritis (*i.e.* body & joint pain), and hayfever (& other allergies), see:

Better Breast Health Naturally with Chinese Medicine, Honora Lee Wolfe, Blue Poppy Press, Boulder, CO, 1998

Curing Arthritis Naturally with Chinese Medicine, Douglas Frank & Bob Flaws, Blue Poppy Press, Boulder, CO, 1997

Curing Depression Naturally with Chinese Medicine, Rosa Schnyer & Bob Flaws, Blue Poppy Press, Boulder, CO, 1998

Curing Hayfever Naturally with Chinese Medicine, Bob Flaws, Blue Poppy Press, Boulder, CO, 1997

Curing Headaches Naturally with Chinese Medicine, Bob Flaws, Blue Poppy Press, Boulder, CO 1998

Curing Insomnia Naturally with Chinese Medicine, Bob Flaws, Blue Poppy Press, Boulder, CO, 1997

Curing Irritable Bowel Syndrome Naturally with Chinese Medicine, Jane Bean Oberski & Bob Flaws, Blue Poppy Press, Boulder, CO, 2000

Curing PMS Naturally with Chinese Medicine, Bob Flaws, Blue Poppy Press, Boulder, CO, 1997

Chinese Medical Glossary

Chinese medicine is a system unto itself. Its technical terms are uniquely its own and cannot be reduced to the definitions of Western medicine without destroying the very fabric and logic of Chinese medicine. Ultimately, because Chinese medicine was created in the Chinese language, Chinese medicine is best and really only understood in that language. Nevertheless, as Westerners trying to understand Chinese medicine, we must translate the technical terms of Chinese medicine in English words. If some of these technical translations sound peculiar at first and their meaning is not immediately apparent, this is because no equivalent concepts exist in everyday English.

In the past, some Western authors have erroneously translated technical Chinese medical terms using Western medical or at least quasi-scientific words in an attempt to make this system more acceptable to Western audiences. For instance, the words tonify and sedate are commonly seen in the Western Chinese medical literature even though, in the case of sedate, its meaning is 180° opposite to the Chinese understanding of the word *xie*. *Xie* means to drain off something which has pooled and accumulated. That accumulation is seen as something excess which should not be lingering where it is. Because it is accumulating somewhere where it shouldn't, it is impeding and obstructing whatever should be moving to and through that area. The word sedate comes from the Latin word *sedere*, to sit. Therefore, the word sedate means to make something sit still. In English, we get the word sediment from this same root. However, the Chinese *xie* means draining off that which is sitting somewhere erroneously. Therefore, to think that one is going to sedate what is already sitting is a great mistake in understanding the clinical implication and application of this technical term.

Therefore, in order to preserve the integrity of this system while still making it intelligible to English language readers, I have appended the following glossary of Chinese medical technical terms. The terms themselves are based on Nigel Wiseman's *English-Chinese Chinese-English Dictionary of Chinese Medicine* published by the Hunan Science & Technology Press in Changsha, People's Republic of China in 1995. Dr. Wiseman is, I believe, the greatest Western scholar in terms of the translation of Chinese medicine into English. As a Chinese reader myself, although I often find Wiseman's terms awkward sounding at first, I also think they convey most accurately the Chinese understanding and logic of these terms.

Acquired essence: Essence manufactured out of the surplus of qi and blood in turn created out of the refined essence of food and drink

Acupoints: Those places on the channels and network vessels where qi and blood tend to collect in denser concentrations, and thus those places where the qi and blood in the channels are especially available for manipulation

Acupuncture: The regulation of qi flow by the stimulation of certain points located on the channels and network vessels achieved mainly by the insertion of fine needles into these points

Aromatherapy: Using various scents and smells to treat and prevent disease

Ascendant hyperactivity of liver yang: Upwardly out of control counterflow of liver yang due to insufficient yin to hold it down in the lower part of the body

Bedroom taxation: Fatigue or vacuity due to excessive sex

Blood: The red colored fluid which flows in the vessels and nourishes and constructs the tissues of the body

Blood stasis: Also called dead blood, malign blood, and dry blood, blood stasis is blood which is no longer moving through the vessels as it should. Instead it is precipitated in the vessels like silt in a river. Like silt, it then obstructs the free flow of the blood in the vessels and also impedes the production of new or fresh blood.

Blood vacuity: Insufficient blood manifesting in diminished nourishment, construction, and moistening of body tissues

Bowels: The hollow yang organs of Chinese medicine

Central qi: Also called the middle qi, this is synonymous with the spleen-stomach qi

Channels: The main routes for the distribution of qi and blood, but mainly qi

Chong & ren: Two of the eight extraordinary vessels which act as reservoirs for all the other channels and vessels of the body. These two govern women's menstruation, reproduction, and lactation in particular.

Clear: The pure or clear part of food and drink ingested which is then turned into qi and blood

Counterflow: An erroneous flow of qi, usually upward but sometimes horizontally as well

Damp heat: A combination of accumulated dampness mixed with pathological heat often associated with sores, abnormal vaginal discharges, and some types of menstrual and body pain

Dampness: A pathological accumulation of body fluids

Decoction: A method of administering Chinese medicinals by boiling these medicinals in water, removing the dregs, and drinking the resulting medicinal liquid

Depression: Stagnation and lack of movement, as in liver depression qi stagnation

Depressive heat: Heat due to enduring or severe qi stagnation which then transforms into heat

Drain: To drain off or away some pathological qi or substance from where it is replete or excess

Essence: A stored, very potent form of substance and qi, usually yin when compared to yang qi, but can be transformed into yang qi

Five phase theory: An ancient Chinese system of correspondences dividing up all of reality into five phases of development which then mutually engender and check each other according to definite sequences

Foot reflexology: The stimulation of zones on the feet which correspond with the viscera and bowels, thus a method of stimulating the internal organs by stimulating the feet

Heat toxins: A particularly virulent and concentrated type of pathological heat often associated with purulence (*i.e.*, pus formation), sores, and sometimes, but not always, malignancies

Heliotherapy: Exposure of the body to sunlight in order to treat and prevent disease

Hydrotherapy: Using various baths and water applications to treat and prevent disease

Lassitude of the spirit: A listless or apathetic affect or emotional demeanor due to obvious fatigue of the mind and body

Life gate fire: Another name for kidney yang or kidney fire, seen as the ultimate source of yang qi in the body

Magnet therapy: Applying magnets to acupuncture points to treat and prevent disease

Moxibustion: Burning the herb Artemisia Argyium on, over, or near acupuncture points in order to add yang qi, warm cold, or promote the movement of the qi and blood

Network vessels: Small vessels which form a net-like web insuring the flow of qi and blood to all body tissues

Phlegm: A pathological accumulation of phlegm or mucus congealed from dampness or body fluids

Portals: Also called orifices, the openings of the sensory organs and the opening of the heart through which the spirit makes contact with the world outside

Qi: Activity, function, that which moves, transforms, defends, restrains, and warms

Qi mechanism: The process of transforming yin substance controlled and promoted by the qi, largely synonymous with the process of digestion

Qi vacuity: Insufficient qi manifesting in diminished movement, transformation, and function

Repletion: A state of fullness, abundance, or exuberance, almost always pathological

Seven star hammer: A small hammer with needles embedded in its head used to stimulate acupoints without actually inserting needles

Spirit: The accumulation of qi in the heart which manifests as consciousness, sensory awareness, and mental-emotional function

Stagnation: Non-movement of the qi, lack of free flow, constraint

Supplement: To add to or augment, as in supplementing the qi, blood, yin, or yang

Turbid: The yin, impure, turbid part of food and drink which is sent downward to be excreted as waste

Vacuity: Emptiness or insufficiency, typically of qi, blood, yin, or yang

Vacuity cold: Obvious signs and symptoms of cold due to a lack or insufficiency of yang qi

Vacuity heat: Heat due to hyperactive yang in turn due to insufficient controlling yin

Vessels: The main routes for the distribution of qi and blood, but mainly blood

Viscera: The solid yin organs of Chinese medicine

Yin: In the body, substance and nourishment

Yin vacuity: Insufficient yin substance necessary to nourish, control, and counterbalance yang activity

Yang: In the body, function, movement, activity, transformation

Yang vacuity: Insufficient warming and transforming function giving rise to symptoms of cold in the body

Bibliography

Chinese language sources

Cheng Dan An Zhen Jiu Xuan Ji (Cheng Dan-an's Selected Acupuncture & Moxibustion Works), ed. by Cheng Wei-fen *et al.*, Shanghai Science & Technology Press, Shanghai, 1986

Chu Zhen Zhi Liao Xue (A Study of Acupuncture Treatment), Li Zhong-yu, Sichuan Science & Technology Press, Chengdu, 1990

Dong Yuan Yi Ji (Dong-yuan's Collected Medical Works), ed. by Bao Zheng-fei *et al.*, People's Health & Hygiene Press, Beijing, 1993

Han Ying Chang Yong Yi Xue Ci Hui (Chinese-English Glossary of Commonly Used Medical Terms), Huang Xiao-kai, People's Health & Hygiene Press, Beijing, 1982

Nan Zhi Bing De Liang Fang Miao Fa (Fine Formulas & Miraculous Methods for Difficult to Treat Diseases), Wu Da-zhou & Ge Xiu-ke, Chinese National Medicine & Medicinal Technology Press, 1992

Nei Ke Bing Liang Fang (Fine Formulas for Internal Medicine), He Yuan-lin & Jiang Chang-yun, Yunnan University Press, Kunming, 1991

Shang Hai Lao Zhong Yi Jing Yan Xuan Bian (A Selected Compilation of Shanghai Old Doctors' Experiences), Shanghai Science & Technology Press, Shanghai, 1984

Shi Yong Zhen Jiu Tui Na Zhi Liao Xue (A Study of Practical Acupuncture, Moxibustion & Tui Na Treatments), Xia Zhi-ping, Shanghai College of Chinese Medicine Press, Shanghai, 1990

Xian Zai Nan Zhi Bing Zhong Yi Zhen Liao Xue (A Study of Diagnosis & Treatmnet of Modern, Difficult to Treat Diseases), Wu Jun-yu & Bai Yong-ke, Chinese Medicine Ancient Books Press, Beijing, 1993

Yan De Xin Zhen Zhi Ning Nan Bing Mi Chi (A Secret Satchel of Yan De-xin's Diagnosis & Treatment of Knotty, Difficult to Treat Diseases), Yan De-xin, Literary Press Publishing Co., Shanghai, 1997

Yi Zong Jin Jian (The Golden Mirror of Ancestral Medicine), Wu Qian *et al.*, People's Health & Hygiene Press, Beijing, 1985

173

Yu Xue Zheng Zhi (Static Blood Patterns & Treatments), Zhang Xue-wen, Shanxi Science & Technology Press, Xian, 1986

Zhen Jiu Da Cheng (A Great Compendium of Acupuncture & Moxibustion), Yang Ji-zhou, People's Health & Hygiene Press, Beijing, 1983

Zhen Jiu Xue (A Study of Acupuncture & Moxibustion), Qiu Mao-liang *et al.*, Shanghai Science & Technology Press, Shanghai, 1985

Zhen Jiu Yi Xue (An Easy Study of Acupuncture & Moxibustion), Li Shou-xian, People's Health & Hygiene Press, Beijing, 1990

Zhong Guo Min Jian Cao Yao Fang (Chinese Folk Herbal Medicinal Formulas), Liu Guang-rui & Liu Shao-lin, Sichuan Science & Technology Press, Chengdu, 1992

Zhong Guo Zhen Jiu Chu Fang Xue (A Study of Chinese Acupuncture & Moxibustion Prescriptions), Xiao Shao-qing, Ningxia People's Press, Yinchuan, 1986

Zhong Guo Zhong Yi Mi Fang Da Quan (A Great Compendium of Chinese National Chinese Medical Secret Formulas), ed. by Hu Zhao-ming, Literary Propagation Publishing Company, Shanghai, 1992

Zhong Yi Bing Yin Bing Ji Xue (A Study of Chinese Medical Disease Causes & Disease Mechanisms), Wu Dun- xu, Shanghai College of TCM Press, Shanghai, 1989

Zhong Yi Hu Li Xue (A Study of Chinese Medical Nursing), Lu Su-ying, People's Health & Hygiene Press, Beijing, 1983

Zhong Yi Lin Chuang Ge Ke (Various Clinical Specialties in Chinese Medicine), Zhang En-qin *et al.*, Shanghai College of TCM Press, Shanghai, 1990

Zhong Yi Ling Yan Fang (Efficacious Chinese Medical Formulas), Lin Bin-zhi, Science & Technology Propagation Press, Beijing, 1991

Zhong Yi Miao Yong Yu Yang Sheng (Chinese Medicine Wondrous Uses & Nourishing Life), Ni Qi-lan, Liberation Army Press, Beijing, 1993

Zhong Yi Nei Ke Lin Chuang Shou Ce (*Handbook of Chinese Medicine Internal Medicine*), Xia De-xin, Shanghai Science & Technology Press, Shanghai, 1989

English language sources

Alternative Medicine Guide to Chronic Fatigue, Fibromyalgia and Environmental Illness, Burton Goldberg, Future Medicine Publishing, 1998

America Exhausted: Breakthrough Treatments of Fatigue and Fibromyalgia, Edward J. Conley, Vitality Press, 1998

A Barefoot Doctor's Manual, revised & enlarged edition, Cloudburst Press, Mayne Isle, 1977

Betrayal of the Brain: The Neurologic Basis of Chronic Fatigue Syndrome, Fibromyalgia Syndrome, and Related Neural Network Disorders, Jay A. Goldstein, Haworth Press, 1996

Chinese-English Manual of Common-used Prescriptions in TraditionaChinese Medicine, Ou Ming, ed., Joint Publishing Co., Ltd., Hong Kong, 1989

Chinese Herbal Medicine: Formulas & Strategies, Dan Bensky & Randall Barolet, Eastland Press, Seattle, 1990

Chinese Self-massage: The Easy Way to health, Fan Ya-li, Blue PoppyPress, Boulder, CO, 1996

A Clinical Guide to Chinese Herbs and Formulae, Cheng Song-yu & Li Fei, Churchill & Livingstone, Edinburgh, 1993

Chinese-English Terminology of Traditional Chinese Medicine, Shuai Xue-zhong *et al.*, Hunan Science & Technology Press, Changsha, 1983

A Compendium of TCM Patterns & Treatments, Bob Flaws & Daniel Finney, Blue Poppy Press, Boulder, CO, 1996

A Comprehensive Guide to Chinese Herbal Medicine, Chen Ze-lin & Chen Mei-fang, Oriental Healing Arts Institute, Long Beach, CA, 1992

175

English-Chinese Chinese-English Dictionary of Chinese Medicine, Nigel Wiseman, Hunan Science & Technology Press, Changsha, 1995

"FMS: Fibromyalgia Syndrome," Devin J. Starlanyl, www.sover.net/~devstar/fmsdef.htm

Fibromyalgia Advocate: Getting the Support You Need to Cope with Fibromyalgia and Myofascial Pain Syndrome, Devin J. Starlanyl, New Harbinger Press, Oakland, CA, 1998

A Handbook of Differential Diagnosis with Key Signs & Symptoms, Therapeutic Principles, and Guiding Prescriptions, Ou-yang Yi, trans. by C. S. Cheung, Harmonious Sunshine Cultural Center, San Francisco, 1987

"A Guide for Patients with Fibromyalgia Syndrome," David A. Nye, Sept. 21, 1997, http://prairie.lakes.com/~roseleaf/fibro/pt-faq.html

A Manual of Acupuncture, Peter Deadman and Mazin Al-Khafaji with Kevin Baker, Journal of Chinese Medicine Publications, Hove, England, 1998

A Practical Dictionary of Chinese Medicine, second edition, Nigel Wiseman and Feng Ye, Paradigm Publications, Brookline, MA, 1998

A Practical English-Chinese Library of Traditional Chinese Medicine: Chinese Massage, Zhang Enqin, editor-in-chief, Publishing House of Shanghai College of TCM, Shanghai, 1988

A Practical English-Chinese Library of Traditional Chinese Medicine: Health Preservation and Rehabilitation, Zhang Enqin, editor- in-chief, Publishing House of Shanghai College of TCM, Shanghai, 1988

Chinese Herbal Medicine: Materia Medica, Dan Bensky & Andrew Gamble, second, revised edition, Eastland Press, Seattle, 1993

Chinese Self-massage: The Easy Way to Health, Fan Ya-li, Blue Poppy Press, Boulder, CO, 1996

"Fibromyalgia: An Age-old Malady Begging for Respect," R. Powers, *Journal of General Internal Medicine,* #8, 1993, p. 93-105

176

Fibromyalgia and Chronic Myofascial Pain Syndrome, Devin J. Starlanyl & Mary Ellen Copeland, New Harbinger Press, Oakland, CA, 1996

"Fibromyalgia: The Copenhagen Declaration," C. Csillag, *Lancet*, #340, 1992, p. 663-664

"Fibromyalgia Syndrome: An Emerging But Controversial Condition," D. L. Goldenberg, *Journal of the American Medical Association (JAMA)*, #257, 1987, p. 2782-2787

Fundamentals of Chinese Acupuncture, Andrew Ellis, Nigel Wiseman & Ken Boss, Paradigm Publications, Brookline, MA, 1988

Fundamentals of Chinese Medicine, Nigel Wiseman & Andrew Ellis, Paradigm Publications, Brookline, MA, 1985

Glossary of Chinese Medical Terms and Acupuncture Points, Nigel Wiseman & Ken Boss, Paradigm Publications, Brookline, MA, 1990

Handbook of Chinese Herbs and Formulas, Him-che Yeung, self-published, CA, 1985

Oriental Materia Medica: A Concise Guide, Hong-yen Hsu, Oriental Healing Arts Institute, Long Beach, CA, 1986

Outline Guide to Chinese Herbal Patent Medicines in Pill Form, Margaret A. Naeser, Boston Chinese Medicine, Boston, MA, 1990

Practical Traditional Chinese Medicine & Pharmacology: Clinical Experiences, Shang Xian-min *et al.*, New World Press, Beijing, 1990

Practical Traditional Chinese Medicine & Pharmacology: Herbal Formulas, Geng Jun-ying, *et al.*, New World Press, Beijing, 1991

The Essential Book of Traditional Chinese Medicine, Vol. 2: Clinical Practice, Liu Yan-chi, trans. by Fang Ting-yu & Chen Lai-di, Columbia University Press, NY, 1988

The Fibromyalgia Help Book, Jenny Fransen & I. Jon Russell, Smith House Press, St. Paul, MN, 1996

The Fibromyalgia Survivor, Mark Pellegrino, Anadem Publishing, Columbus, OH, 1996

The Merck Manual of Diagnosis & Therapy, 15th edition, ed. by Robert Berkow, Merck Sharp & Dohme Research Laboratories, Rahway, NJ, 1987

The Nanjing Seminars Transcript, Qiu Mao-lian & Su Xu-ming, The Journal of Chinese Medicine, UK, 1985

The Practice of Chinese Medicine: The Treatment of Diseases with Acupuncture and Chinese Herbs, Giovanni Maciocia, Churchill Livingstone, Edinburgh, 1994

"The Prevalence and Characteristics of Fibromyalgia in the General Population," F. Wolfe, K. Ross, *et al.*, *Arthritis & Rheumatology*, #38, 1995, p. 19-28

The Treatise on the Spleen & Stomach, Li Dong-yuan, trans. by Yang Shou-zhong, Blue Poppy Press, Boulder, CO, 1993

The Treatment of Disease in TCM, Volume 1: Diseases of the Head and Face Including Mental / Emotional Disorders, Philippe Sionneau and Lü Gang, Blue Poppy Press, Boulder, CO, 1996

The Yeast Connection, William G. Crook, Vintage Books, Random House, NY, 1986

The Yeast Syndrome, John Parks Towbridge & Morton Walker, Bantam Books, Toronto, 1988

Traditional Medicine in Contemporary China, Nathan Sivin, University of Michigan, Ann Arbor, 1987

Zang Fu: The Organ Systems of Traditional Chinese Medicine, second edition, Jeremy Ross, Churchill Livingstone, Edinburgh, 1985

Index

A

abdominal cramping 60, 72, 147
abdominal distention 52, 59
abdominal fullness 30
abdominal pain 63, 72, 109, 121, 125, 127, 128, 147, 148
acupuncture v, 24, 48, 49, 61, 62, 87-90, 92-95, 97, 114, 122, 123, 125, 128, 134, 135, 138, 145, 155-157, 159-161, 163, 164, 168, 170, 173, 174, 176-178
aerobic exercise 106, 108
age spots 54
agitation 16, 24, 42, 92, 141
alcohol 89, 100, 102-105, 135, 137
allergic rhinitis 5, 57
allergies 4, 15, 56, 81, 93, 103-105, 155, 165, 166
allergies, respiratory 56
An Shen Bu Xin Wan 77
anger 18, 21, 43, 109, 110, 112
anger, easy 109
antibiotic use 104
antidepressants 6
anus, burning around the 60, 79
anxiety 24, 54, 92, 117, 118, 141
anxiousness 42
appetite, loss of 21, 52
arthritis, rheumatoid 1, 2
aromatherapy, Chinese 117, 118
asthma 5, 56, 57, 62, 81

B

Ba Zheng San Wan 71
belching 52
bladder infections, recurrent 104
bleeding, abnormal 52, 75
blindness, night 5, 54
bloating 4, 21, 30, 79
bloating after meals 21, 79
body pain, generalized 3, 11
bowel function 48
bowel movements, cramping before 60
bowel movements, increased number of 52
breast distention & pain 150
breast distention and pain 44, 52, 72, 150
breast disease, fibrocystic 6, 56, 155, 166
breath, shortness of 56
bruising, easy 15, 52, 59
bruxism 93
Bu Zhong Yi Qi Wan 80
burping and belching 52

C

calisthenics 107
candidiasis 103, 165
chapped lips 53
cherry hemangiomas 54
Chinese Self-massage Therapy: The Easy Way to Health 122
clear, bland diet 101, 105, 165
coffee 102, 104, 118
cold extremities 4
cold lower half of the body 55
constipation 5, 52-54, 63, 72, 109, 121, 125, 127-129, 132, 144, 147-149, 151, 152
constipation, fluid dryness 152
cooked meals 114
coordination, poor 119
counterflow qi 128
cramping 4, 60, 72, 109, 147
cravings, chocolate 102

D

Da Bu Yin Wan 82
Dan Zhi Xiao Yao Wan 74
deep relaxation 62, 97, 109-115, 117, 163
depression iii, v, 2, 5, 7, 11, 19, 22, 35, 37-39, 41, 43-45, 51, 52, 55, 59-63, 65, 66, 68, 69, 72-74, 77, 82, 88, 90, 91, 94, 102-105, 109, 110, 112, 117-120, 122, 127, 132, 137, 138, 141, 142, 144, 146, 147, 150, 155, 166, 169

T

tension headaches 120
*The Book of Jook: Chinese Medicinal
    Porridges* 152, 165
Tian Wang Bu Xin Dan 76
Tong Xie Yao Fang 72
tongue, black and blue marks on the
    54
tongue, pale 54, 55, 75
tremors 6

U, V, W

unrest 16, 24, 74
urinary capacity, decreased 5
urinary incontinence 15
urination, burning 62
urination, frequent 55, 133
urination, nighttime 26, 54, 119,
    139, 142
urination, scanty, darkish 54
uterine bleeding, abnormal 52
uterine prolapse 15
vacuity taxation 11
varicosities 54, 61
vision, blurred 4, 5, 7, 54
vomiting 34, 121
weakness 20, 21, 26, 55, 80, 100,
    119, 142

X, Y

Xanax 6
Xiang Sha Liu Jun Zi Wan 68, 79
Xiao Feng San Wan 67
Xiao Yao Wan 72, 74
yeast infections 104
Yi Guan Jian Wan 81
yin and yang 12-14, 19, 25, 26, 43,
    46, 48, 62, 78, 84
Yu Ping Feng San Wan 81

OTHER BOOKS ON CHINESE MEDICINE AVAILABLE FROM BLUE POPPY PRESS

3450 Penrose Place, Suite 110, Boulder, CO 80301
For ordering 1-800-487-9296 PH. 303\447-8372 FAX 303\245-8362
Email: bpeinc1@cs.com Website: www.bluepoppy.com

A NEW AMERICAN ACUPUNCTURE by Mark Seem, ISBN 0-936185-44-9

ACUPOINT POCKET REFERENCE ISBN 0-936185-93-7

ACUPUNCTURE AND MOXIBUSTION FORMULAS & TREATMENTS by Cheng Dan-an, trans. by Wu Ming, ISBN 0-936185-68-6

ACUPUNCTURE PHYSICAL MEDICINE: An Acupuncture Touchpoint Approach to the Treatment of Chronic Pain, Fatigue, and Stress Disorders by Mark Seem ISBN 1-891845-13-6

ACUTE ABDOMINAL SYNDROMES: Diagnosis & Treatment by Combined Chinese-Western Med. by Alon Marcus, ISBN 0-936185-31-7

AGING & BLOOD STASIS: A New Approach to TCM Geriatrics by Yan De-xin, ISBN 0-936185-63-5

AIDS & ITS TREATMENT ACCORDING TO TRADITIONAL CHINESE MEDICINE by Huang Bing-shan, trans. by Fu-Di & Bob Flaws, ISBN 0-936185-28-7

BETTER BREAST HEALTH NATURALLY with CHINESE MEDICINE by Honora Lee Wolfe & Bob Flaws ISBN 0-936185-90-2

THE BOOK OF JOOK: Chinese Medicinal Porridges, An Alternative to the Typical Western Breakfast by B. Flaws, ISBN0-936185-60-0

CHINESE MEDICAL PALMISTRY: Your Health in Your Hand by Zong Xiao-fan & Gary Liscum, ISBN 0-936185-64-3

CHINESE MEDICINAL TEAS: Simple, Proven, Folk Formulas for Common Diseases & Promoting Health by Zong Xiao-fan & Gary Liscum, ISBN 0-936185-76-7

CHINESE MEDICINAL WINES & ELIXIRS Bob Flaws, ISBN 0-936185-58-9

CHINESE PEDIATRIC MASSAGE THERAPY: A Parent's & Practitioner's Guide to the Prevention & Treatment of Childhood Illness by Fan Ya-li, ISBN 0-936185-54-6

CHINESE SELF-MASSAGE THERAPY: The Easy Way to Health by Fan Ya-li ISBN 0-936185-74-0

THE CLASSIC OF DIFFICULTIES: A Translation of the *Nan Jing* ISBN 1-891845-07-1

A COMPENDIUM OF TCM PATTERNS & TREATMENTS by Bob Flaws & Daniel Finney, ISBN 0-936185-70-8

CURING ARTHRITIS NATURALLY WITH CHINESE MEDICINE by Douglas Frank & Bob Flaws ISBN 0-936185-87-2

CURING DEPRESSION NATURALLY WITH CHINESE MEDICINE by Rosa Schnyer & Bob Flaws ISBN 0-936185-94-5

CONTROLLING DIABETES NATURALLY WITH CHINESE MEDICINE by Lynn Kuchinski ISBN 1-891845-06-3

CURING HAY FEVER NATURALLY WITH CHINESE MEDICINE by Bob Flaws, ISBN 0-936185-91-0

CURING HEADACHES NATURALLY WITH CHINESE MEDICINE, by Bob Flaws, ISBN 0-936185-95-3-X

CURING IBS NATURALLY WITH CHINESE MEDICINE, by Jane Bean Oberski, ISBN 1-891845-11-X

CURING INSOMNIA NATURALLY WITH CHINESE MEDICINE by Bob Flaws ISBN 0-936185-85-6

CURING PMS NATURALLY WITH CHINESE MEDICINE by Bob Flaws ISBN 0-936185-85-6

A STUDY OF DAOIST ACUPUNCTURE & MOXIBUSTION by Liu Zheng-cai ISBN 1-891845-08-X

THE DIVINE FARMER'S MATERIA MEDICA (*A Translation of the Shen Nong Ben Cao*) ISBN 0-936185-96-1

THE DIVINELY RESPONDING CLASSIC: A Translation of the Shen Ying Jing from Zhen Jiu Da Cheng, trans. by Yang Shou-zhong & Liu Feng-ting ISBN 0-936185-55-4

DUI YAO: THE ART OF COMBINING CHINESE HERBAL MEDICINALS by Philippe Sionneau ISBN 0-936185-81-3

ENDOMETRIOSIS, INFERTILITY AND TRADITIONAL CHINESE MEDICINE: A Laywoman's Guide by Bob Flaws ISBN 0-936185-14-7

THE ESSENCE OF LIU FENG-WU'S GYNECOLOGY by Liu Feng-wu, translated by Yang Shou-zhong ISBN 0-936185-88-0

EXTRA TREATISES BASED ON INVESTIGATION & INQUIRY: A Translation of Zhu Dan-xi's Ge Zhi Yu Lun, by Yang & Duan, ISBN 0-936185-53-8

FIRE IN THE VALLEY: TCM Diagnosis & Treatment of Vaginal Diseases ISBN 0-936185-25-2

FU QING-ZHU'S GYNECOLOGY trans. by Yang Shou-zhong and Liu Da-wei, ISBN 0-936185-35-X

FULFILLING THE ESSENCE: A Handbook of Traditional & Contemporary Treatments for Female Infertility by Bob Flaws, ISBN 0-936185-48-1

GOLDEN NEEDLE WANG LE-TING: A 20th Century Master's Approach to Acupuncture by Yu Hui-chan and Han Fu-ru, trans. by Shuai Xue-zhong

A HANDBOOK OF TRADITIONAL CHINESE DERMATOLOGY by Liang Jian-hui, trans. by Zhang & Flaws, ISBN 0-936185-07-4

A HANDBOOK OF TRADITIONAL CHINESE GYNECOLOGY by Zhejiang College of TCM, trans. by Zhang Ting-liang, ISBN 0-936185-06-6 (4th edit.)

A HANDBOOK OF MENSTRUAL DISEASES IN CHINESE MEDICINE by Bob Flaws ISBN 0-936185-82-1

A HANDBOOK of TCM PEDIATRICS by Bob Flaws, ISBN 0-936185-72-4

A HANDBOOK OF TCM UROLOGY & MALE SEXUAL DYSFUNCTION by Anna Lin, OMD, ISBN 0-936185-36-8

THE HEART & ESSENCE OF DAN-XI'S METHODS OF TREATMENT by Xu Dan-xi, trans. by Yang, ISBN 0-926185-49-X

THE HEART TRANSMISSION OF MEDICINE by Liu Yi-ren, trans. by Yang Shou-zhong ISBN 0-936185-83-X

HIGHLIGHTS OF ANCIENT ACUPUNCTURE PRESCRIPTIONS trans. by Wolfe & Crescenz ISBN 0-936185-23-6

HOW TO WRITE A TCM HERBAL FORMULA: A Logical Methodology for the Formulation & Administration of Chinese Herbal Medicine in Decoction by Bob Flaws, ISBN 0-936185-49-X

IMPERIAL SECRETS OF HEALTH & LONGEVITY by Bob Flaws, ISBN 0-936185-51-1

KEEPING YOUR CHILD HEALTHY WITH CHINESE MEDICINE by Bob Flaws, ISBN 0-936185-71-6

THE LAKESIDE MASTER'S STUDY OF THE PULSE by Li Shi-zhen, trans. by Bob Flaws, ISBN 1-891845-01-2

Li Dong-yuan's TREATISE ON THE SPLEEN & STOMACH, *A Translation of the Pi Wei Lun* by Yang & Li, ISBN 0-936185-41-4

LOW BACK PAIN: Care & Prevention with Chinese Medicine by Douglas Frank, ISBN 0-936185-66-X

MASTER HUA'S CLASSIC OF THE CENTRAL VISCERA by Hua Tuo, ISBN 0-936185-43-0

MASTER TONG'S ACUPUNCTURE: An Ancient Alternative Style in Modern Clinical Practice by Miriam Lee 0-926185-37-6

THE MEDICAL I CHING: Oracle of the Healer Within by Miki Shima, OMD, ISBN 0-936185-38-4

MANAGING MENOPAUSE NATURALLY with Chinese Medicine by Honora Wolfe ISBN 0-936185-98-8

PAO ZHI: Introduction to Processing Chinese Medicinals to Enhance Their Therapeutic Effect, by Philippe Sionneau, ISBN 0-936185-62-1

PATH OF PREGNANCY, VOL. I, Gestational Disorders by Bob Flaws, ISBN 0-936185-39-2

PATH OF PREGNANCY, Vol. II, Postpartum Diseases by Bob Flaws. ISBN 0-936185-42-2

PEDIATRIC BRONCHITIS: Its Cause, Diagnosis & Treatment According to TCM trans. by Gao Yu-li and Bob Flaws, ISBN 0-936185-26-0

PRINCE WEN HUI'S COOK: Chinese Dietary Therapy by Bob Flaws & Honora Lee Wolfe, ISBN 0-912111-05-4, $12.95 (Published by Paradigm Press)

THE PULSE CLASSIC: A Translation of the *Mai Jing* by Wang Shu-he, trans. by Yang Shou-zhong ISBN 0-936185-75-9

SEVENTY ESSENTIAL TCM FORMULAS FOR BEGINNERS by Bob Flaws, ISBN 0-936185-59-7

SHAOLIN SECRET FORMULAS for Treatment of External Injuries, by De Chan, ISBN 0-936185-08-2

STATEMENTS OF FACT IN TRADITIONAL CHINESE MEDICINE by Bob Flaws, ISBN 0-936185-52-X

STICKING TO THE POINT 1: A Rational Methodology for the Step by Step Formulation & Administration of an Acupuncture Treatment by Bob Flaws ISBN 0-936185-17-1

STICKING TO THE POINT 2: A Study of Acupuncture & Moxibustion Formulas and Strategies by Bob Flaws ISBN 0-936185-97-X

A STUDY OF DAOIST ACUPUNCTURE by Liu Zheng-cai ISBN 1-891845-08-X

TEACH YOURSELF TO READ MODERN MEDICAL CHINESE by Bob Flaws, ISBN 0-936185-99-6

THE SYSTEMATIC CLASSIC OF ACUPUNCTURE & MOXIBUSTION (*Jia Yi Jing*) by Huang-fu Mi, trans. by Yang Shou-zhong & Charles Chace, ISBN 0-936185-29-5

THE TAO OF HEALTHY EATING ACCORDING TO CHINESE MEDICINE by Bob Flaws, ISBN 0-936185-92-9

THE TREATMENT OF DISEASE IN TCM, Vol I: Diseases of the Head & Face Including Mental/Emotional Disorders by Philippe Sionneau & Lü Gang, ISBN 0-936185-69-4

THE TREATMENT OF DISEASE IN TCM, Vol. II: Diseases of the Eyes, Ears, Nose, & Throat by Sionneau & Lü, ISBN 0-936185-69-4

THE TREATMENT OF DISEASE, Vol. III: Diseases of the Mouth, Lips, Tongue, Teeth & Gums, by Sionneau & Lü, ISBN 0-936185-79-1

THE TREATMENT OF DISEASE, Vol IV: Diseases of the Neck, Shoulders, Back, & Limbs, by Philippe Sionneau & Lü Gang, ISBN 0-936185-89-9

THE TREATMENT OF DISEASE, Vol V: Diseases of the Chest & Abdomen, by Philippe Sionneau & Lü Gang, ISBN 1-891845-02-0

THE TREATMENT OF DISEASE, Vol VI: Diseases of the Urogential System & Proctology, by Philippe Sionneau & Lü Gang, ISBN 1-891845-05-5

THE TREATMENT OF EXTERNAL DISEASES WITH ACUPUNCTURE & MOXIBUSTION by Yan Cui-lan and Zhu Yun-long, ISBN 0-936185-80-5

160 ESSENTIAL CHINESE HERBAL PATENT MEDICINES by Bob Flaws ISBN 1-891945-12-8

630 QUESTIONS & ANSWERS ABOUT CHINESE HERBAL MEDICINE: a Workbook & Study Guide by Bob Flaws ISBN 1-891845-04-7

230 ESSENTIAL CHINESE MEDICINALS by Bob Flaws, ISBN 1-891845-03-9p